The

Holistic Guide

To

Twin Pregnancy

BreAnn Blehm

BreAnn Blehm

Dedication

To Daddy.
For always believing.
For always encouraging.
For all the big dreams.

Table of Contents

Holistic: adjective:

1: identifying with principles of holism in a system of therapeutics, especially one considered outside the mainstream of scientific medicine...often involving nutritional measures.

2: study of a person as a whole, and not just the sum of their parts.

Welcome

"Being a mother of twins is learning about strengths you didn't know you had and dealing with fears you didn't know existed."

Unknown

Congratulations! If you are reading this Guide to Twin Pregnancy then more than likely, you are expecting twins. Or you just have an interesting taste in reading material. This is an incredible journey that opens a new chapter in your life. It won't always be easy, or pretty, and the emotions that come with it will take their toll. However, there are two beautiful babies waiting for you at the end of it and I promise it's worth every ache, pain, and stretch mark.

When I first started doing research on what to expect with twin pregnancy, everyone and everything said the same scary words over and over. High risk. Preterm labor. Automatic C-Section. Premature babies. NICU. Being holistically minded, I refused to accept these things as an expected part of my pregnancy. There had to be another way. There had to be a natural approach to twin pregnancy that did not end with me being cut open and my preterm babies whisked away to an incubator for an untold length of time.

In the weeks after finding out that I was expecting twins, I became a sponge. I read everything I could get my hands on. I read first-hand accounts and medical journals. I read theories, ideas, and experimental studies. I studied statistics, methods, standard procedures and practices. I searched high and low for information that would help me make the best and healthiest choices for my body and my growing babies. I was relentless in my pursuit to bring healthy twins earth side so they could begin life with the best start possible, and I am happy to say that I achieved it. My twins were born full term, weighing in at 6 pounds and 9 ounces each. They were healthy and perfect, and required no time in the NICU. I delivered them at a stand-alone birth center with no medical intervention (in fact, Twin A was born in the front seat of our truck in a parking lot…more on that later). We were able to take our babies home the same day we had them.

I wrote this book with the intention of sharing my own twin pregnancy experience, as well as the wealth of information I learned along the way. There are many people who think I simply got lucky; that delivering healthy, full-term twins was the equivalent of winning the lottery. However, I credit the choices I made and the holistic outlook I had with my pregnancy for our positive pregnancy experience and delivery. I whole-heartedly believe that a conscientious approach to your pregnancy, with special attention on prenatal care, support and nutrition can make a difference in the outcome. I simply want to shine a light for other women walking this now familiar road, with an emphasis on the holistic and natural viewpoint.

Official Disclaimer: I am not a doctor. I am not licensed to give medical advice and I certainly am not advocating that you abandon your current doctor or method of medical care. I will share my personal experiences and research with you, but at no point should it ever replace common sense or the advice of your chosen medical professional. I hope this book will do a lot of things for you, but it will not deliver your babies.

Thank you for reading, and welcome to the Twin Mama Club.

Chapter 1

Twins 101

"There are two things in life for which we are never truly prepared: twins."

Josh Billings

"Are they twins?"

"Are they identical?"

"Do twins run in your family?"

"Were they planned?"

"Can you tell them apart?"

"I always wanted twins!"

"My cousin's sister had twins."

"I bet you don't sleep!"

"Were they conceived naturally, or did you have IVF?"

"You've got your hands full!"

These are just a few of the questions and comments you will encounter from well-meaning strangers as you venture into the public with your twins. Babies in general tend to catch the attention of random people; their smooth skin, bright eyes, and overall newness acts like a beacon to the world around them. However, two babies seem to be an irresistible invitation to conversation that ranges from mundane to slightly invasive. It can be overwhelming to encounter, especially when a quick trip to the grocery store for bread and eggs turns into an hour-long endeavor as you field the same questions over and over from curious onlookers. All the attention can leave you feeling like either a Rockstar, or a circus side show. However, as annoying as it can potentially be, I've found their interest is genuine. People are simply fascinated by twins, and for good reason.

Historically, twins were a rare occurrence. Their births were either viewed as a sign of luck or an omen, depending on the surrounding culture. In Greek mythology, twins were thought to be a result of conception from a god. The famous Greek twins Apollo and Artemis, the sun god and the moon goddess, were a reflection of the opposing sides of nature. Twins were believed to be two parts of one whole, each completing the other and neither one quite as powerful on their own as when united. The Greek twins Castor and Pollux embody the deep and powerful bond that twins are said to share. In the mythology, Castor dies and Pollux sacrifices half of his immortality to be with his brother, believing that he could not continue living with half a soul. Zeus granted his wish and cast Castor and Pollux into the night sky as the now famous Gemini constellation.

In many cultures, twins were believed to be mortal enemies with one embracing "good" and the other embracing "evil", each with a predisposed destiny to defeat the other. The good versus evil twins is a common theme in many mythologies across history, and this idea has trickled down through the ages. Everything from Shakespeare to modern day film has utilized the good twin/evil twin storyline.

In West Africa, twins are believed to be supernatural beings. They are termed as spirit children due to their connection to the supernatural world. These spirit children are believed to be capable of bringing either great fortune or great disappointment to their families. They also believe that the twin that is born first is actually the younger of the two, as the eldest is the more important and as such, sends the younger forth to prepare the way. Other variations of this belief are that the elder twin remains in the womb to help guide the younger one out first.

Chinese culture views twins as a sign of good fortune. Images of the Hehe Erxian, or laughing twins, is commonly seen in wedding celebrations to usher forth luck. The laughing twins are said to be immortal Tao monks, who may or may not have been real historical figures during the Tang dynasty.

Today, unlike historical times past, twins are no longer rare. In 2014, the twin birth rate hit a record high according to the Center for Disease Control, with twin births accounting for 33 births out of every 1000. As romantic as the notion of twins being born of gods and supernatural interferences is, science has a different conclusion for the increasing occurrence. First, the use of invitro fertilization has greatly impacted the twin birth rate. Since the introduction of IVF in 1980, the twin birth rate has grown by almost 75%. This is due in part to the emotional and financial cost of IVF. Many couples decide to implant multiple viable embryos in hopes of increasing their chances of conception. However, IVF isn't solely responsible for the twin boom. One study indicates that women are waiting longer to have children, and as result are getting pregnant over the age of 35. Women over 35 have a greater tendency to conceive twins as their bodies make a hormone that stimulates egg production, resulting in the release of more than one egg per ovulation cycle.

Causations of Twinning:

Twins are the result when one of two things happen. Either A) one egg is split into two separate embryos after being fertilized by one sperm which produces identical (or if you want to impress your friends by being super technical: monozygotic) twins; or B) a woman ovulates two separate eggs that are then fertilized by two separate sperm resulting in fraternal (dizygotic) twins. For those who undergo IVF, two separate eggs are fertilized by two separate sperm leading to fraternal twins; though it is still possible for one egg to split to form identical twins after being placed into the uterus.

Identical (monozygotic) twins are almost always of the same gender, as a result of splitting from one egg and sperm, and are genetically considered almost completely identical, save for a few factors like fingerprints. They have identical blood groups, and usually favor each other both physically and emotionally. Identical twins account for almost one third of all twin births. It is extremely rare, but possible, for identical twins to be of separate genders; however, this is a result of a chromosomal abnormality in which there is an extra x chromosome. It is so rare that there have only been 10 cases ever recorded of this happening. Turner Syndrome, also extremely rare, is another instance that would cause monozygotic twins to be of different genders. Both of these chromosomal incidences are so rare that it is almost universally accepted that identical twins are of the same gender. Famous examples of identical twins include Drew and Jonathan Scott of hit HGTV show The Property Brothers, and Mary-Kate and Ashley Olsen.

Fraternal (dizygotic) twins can be the same or different genders, but their genetic composition is no more similar than that of any other set of siblings. As there were two eggs and two sperm involved in creating fraternal twins, as is the case with any singleton, they are simply considered to be siblings that just happened to be born at the same time. They may look alike, they may not. They may have the same chromosomal make-up, but it's more than likely that they won't. My twins are fraternal, a boy and a girl, and not only do they look nothing alike, but they are also very different in regard to personality. They are no more alike to each other than they are to their older brother. Famous examples of fraternal twins include Scarlett Johansson and her brother Hunter, and Ashton Kutcher and his brother Michael.

It Runs in the Family:

There is a common misconception that somehow your likelihood of having twins is dependent on whether or not it "runs in your family". You will be asked by friends and strangers alike whether an aunt, mother, grandmother, great grandmother, etc…passed the "twin gene" on to you. I'm sorry to be the one to say that it doesn't really work like that.

Identical twins are believed to be a spontaneous and random event within the uterus that is not influenced by outside factors such as genetics. That's a nice way of saying that we have no idea why a fertilized egg splits into two embryos after conception. Therefore, this type of twinning does not run in the family. A close male family friend that I grew up with had a grandmother who had an identical twin. He and his wife went on to conceive identical twins and his female cousin, within the same maternal genes, also conceived identical twins. While it may seem a bit extreme to believe there is no correlation between the three sets of identical twins that occurred within three generations of the same family, there is no science at this time that can provide evidence that there is a genetic link. In this particular example, there would have to have been a genetic trait passed through my male friend that also passed through his female cousin that somehow resulted in identical twins. However, studies that have been done in this area cannot find anything in the sperm that would force an egg to separate after fertilization, nor is there any genetic trait that leads scientists to believe that a female has any control over whether or not an egg splits into two (or more) embryos after fertilization. Maybe two grandchildren of an identical twin having identical twins is all simply a coincidence, or maybe there is so much more to discover regarding the science and causes of monozygotic twins. Maybe one day, science will have an answer as to why an egg splits to form two babies. Or maybe, it really is a supernatural occurrence and the world simply needed two of these precious souls.

When it comes to fraternal twins, however, studies have shown that it is possible that hyper-ovulation (ovulating more than one egg at a time) might be a result of genetics passed through the mother, thus increasing the incidence of fraternal twins within a family line. This genetic link to the hyper-ovulation tendency would explain why the granddaughter of a fraternal twin might go on to conceive fraternal twins as well. This genetic link is only passed through the mother, however, so despite what Greek mythology suggests, the male sperm has nothing to do with whether or not multiple babies result out of a single pregnancy. The notion that twins are a result of the prowess and virility of the father is simply a myth born of cultures that place superiority and higher importance on the role that the father has in procreation. My own family history is pretty much devoid of twins, save for a set produced by my paternal great-aunt, so while it is possible for fraternal twins to be passed genetically from one generation to the next, there is no indication that I was genetically predisposed to conceive twins. This leads me to believe that my hyper-ovulation was a result of hormones as I was still nursing my first when I conceived my twins, or an unknown environmental factor. As is the case with identical twins, when it comes to causation of fraternal twins there is still so much that science has yet to unveil. It will be interesting to see what we discover in this realm in the coming years, especially as the incidences of twins continues to rise.

Twin Pregnancy Types:

While the various differences of identical and fraternal twins may seem irrelevant to you now, establishing which type you are carrying is helpful in determining the risks you may encounter, as not every twin pregnancy is the same. There are three main types of twin pregnancy: Dichorionic/Diamniotic, Monochorionic/diamniotic, and monochorionic/monoamniotic. When spoken, words like dichorionic, diamniotic monoamniotic, and monochorionic sound incredibly fancy but when you break it down it becomes a little more self-explanatory. Mono is simply a prefix meaning "one", and Di is a prefix meaning "two". Amniotic refers to the sacs/fluids, while chorionic refers to the Human Chorionic Gonadotropin (hCG) or Chorionic villi, which is essentially pieces of placental tissue that help create your babies genetic build. In this particular context the use of chorionic is in reference to the placenta. To translate into understandable terms, you are either carrying two placentas and two sacs (dichorionic/diamniotic), one placenta and two sacs (monochorionic/diamniotic), or one placenta and one sac (Monochorionic/monoamniotic).

Many times, determining the type of twins you have can be done by ultrasound. A qualified technician can tell whether or not each baby is in its own sac and they may also be able to determine if there is more than one placenta, if the ultrasound is done before the placentas have had a chance to fuse, thus creating the illusion of only one placenta. Your pregnancy type is also an indication of whether your twins are fraternal or identical.

In a Dichorionic/Diamniotic (Di/Di) pregnancy each baby has their own amniotic sac and their own placenta. Fraternal twins are always Di/Di, as they are a result of two eggs being fertilized by two sperm. Each fertilized egg creates its own sac and placenta to support the baby. It is possible for monozygotic twins to be Di/Di, if the split from one fertilized egg and sperm happened no later than 2-3 days after fertilization. While twins in a Di/Di pregnancy have their own placenta, it is not uncommon for the placentas to become fused together as the babies and the placentas grow, with the fusion occurring around the 15th-20th week of pregnancy depending on where the placentas are positioned on the uterine wall. There is not any evidence that fused placentas cause any great risk to twins in utero, because even while fused they are still two separate placentas creating nutrients for each baby. A Di/Di pregnancy is considered to have the lowest risks for both mother and babies. It is also the most common type of pregnancy with spontaneous twins.

In a Monochorionic/Diamniotic (Mo/Di) pregnancy there is one outer sac and one placenta, with each baby having their own inner amniotic sacs. Twins in this type of pregnancy are separated only by the thin membrane of their sacs. Mo/Di pregnancies occur exclusively with identical twins, with one egg and one sperm splitting 3-8 days after fertilization and is the most common pregnancy type among identical twins. Since the twins are sharing a placenta in this scenario, there is a slight increase for risks that you won't see in a Di/Di pregnancy; however, do not let that scare you. Many women with Mo/Di pregnancies go on to have healthy pregnancies and babies. This slight increase of risk is just that: slight. As a result, Mo/Di pregnancies are typically monitored a little more closely than Di/Di and at times, require supervision from a maternal fetal specialist. A maternal fetal specialist has the skills and knowledge to observe an ultrasound and spot any issues that may be occurring. A skilled specialist in this field can help bring peace of mind to you and help manage any irregularities they may find in a positive proactive approach.

In a Monoamniotic/monochorionic (Mo/Mo) pregnancy, there is one inner and outer sac and one placenta that your babies must share. Like, Mo/Di, Mo/Mo twins are always identical. This is considered to be the most high-risk type of twin pregnancy, but it is also one of the rarest. A Mo/Mo pregnancy occurs when one egg is fertilized by one sperm, and splits into two separate eggs 8-13 days after fertilization. If the egg separation occurs any later than 13 days you begin encountering the phenomenon of conjoined twins, which is when the single embryo begins to separate into another but fails to completely disengage from the other before continuing development. Conjoined twins introduce many complications, especially if in their development they share vital main organs like the brain, heart, or liver. This type of pregnancy, which is the rarest of all, is also the most heavily monitored due to the increased potential for complications. That being said, again, please do not let this scare you. I personally know multiple women who have had healthy Mo/Mo pregnancies with healthy babies.

By confirming whether your babies are sharing an amniotic sac or placenta, you will be able to better devise the kind of care you will need as you continue through your pregnancy. A lot of risk can be managed and prevented if the knowledge of its potential existence is there, and this knowledge will help you and your care provider determine the best way to approach your pregnancy both medically and emotionally. Whether you are at the lower end of the risk spectrum with Di/Di twins or the higher end with Mo/Mo twins, know that you can take charge of your health and the health of your babies. As we go through various chapters of this book, I go into more depth regarding risks, and the things you can do that can have a very real impact on your duration of gestation and overall health of your babies. Knowledge is power, and I hope this book fills you with both.

Chapter 2

The Physical Expectations

"Everything grows rounder and wider and weirder, and I sit here in the middle of it all and wonder who in the world you will turn out to be."

Carrie Fisher

Pregnancy in general can be trying. Some women love it, some women hate it. I tend to fall into the former category. Never in my life have I felt like more of a goddess than when I was creating life. I love watching my body grow and feeling my babies wiggle inside me.

My first pregnancy was a beautiful experience, in which I felt like I truly enjoyed every moment. I glowed and stayed active. I grew a cute, loveable bump, and my energy and excitement levels were at an all-time high. However, carrying my twins for nine months was a bittersweet experience. I wanted to love it, and some days I did, but trying to enjoy every moment of my twin pregnancy while it was taking a vast toll on my body and emotions was hard. I wavered between loving it and hating it, with a nice helping of guilt sprinkled in for good measure.

The female body was created to procreate and watching yourself stretch beyond comfort and imagination is truly a magical thing. It is also a very hard thing physically, mentally, and emotionally, and there will be days when it simply feels like it's too much. You will reach a point, fairly quickly, where you feel like your body can't possibly stretch anymore and yet week after week it keeps stretching and growing; turning whatever body you had before pregnancy into nothing more than a home for two humans you haven't even met.

Growing twins is not for the weak. It pushed me to the limits of what I could handle more than anything I've ever gone through in my life. I distinctly remember driving home from the grocery store one day when a sudden and inexplicable urge to pull over and cry hit me. I was tired, and my body ached, and at 20 weeks my stomach was already pushing against the steering wheel, and I was so hungry and nauseous at the same time that it all felt like too much.

I can't do this anymore, I thought weakly, as tears lined my eyes. It was an illogical thought, born out of exhaustion and fear, because let's face it, it's not like I had an alternative option than to keep doing it.

You can do it. You're doing it right now. Look at you doing it. Just keep doing it for another hour. Then eat a snack and take a nap. It will all be okay. The voice in my head was stronger and more confident than I felt in that moment, but I listened to it. Instead of pulling over and crying, I went home and took a nap. Instead of giving in to my fear and exhaustion and listening to that negative voice in my head, I listened to the other voice in my head; the confident, stubborn one that practically annoyed me with its positivity and was capable of ruining a perfectly good pity party. Day by day, I kept doing it. Sometimes, it was an hour by hour type of survival situation, but the more I listened to the positive side of my brain, and pushed out the negative thoughts, the better I became at telling myself "you can do this!" Even on the hard days. Even on the days when I simply wanted to rewind, or fast forward, the clock to a time when there were not two additional people occupying my body.

As much as possible, I tried to look at my pregnancy with a glass half full approach, seeking out the silver linings and clinging to the good things. There were good days and moments with long stretches of time that felt a bit like a normal pregnancy. The second trimester was a bit of a sweet spot for me as the trials and worries of the first trimester had started to ease up and I was still feeling comfortable enough to get up and out a bit despite my rapidly growing bump. I used this trimester to savor the time with my toddler as an only child and to accomplish what I could while my energy was high, my morning sickness low, and my body still manageable to navigate through daily life. I tried hard to take advantage of the good days while I had them in an effort to love this pregnancy, and to carry me through the bad days when love wasn't my primary emotion.

There were beautiful things about carrying twins that I will always remember with fondness, moments that feel like warm rays of sunshine in a rainy season. The sheer amount of movement radiating throughout my body was amazing and surreal. I loved getting to feel my babies move and I came to know each of them by their kicks and soft rolls. When movement would ripple across my belly, I was usually fairly certain which twin was the one stretching and kicking. Baby A was rooted pretty firmly into my pelvis, and all movement lower in my body (and against my bladder) was from his arms and legs reaching out. Baby B was high up under my ribs, with her head nestled close to her brother's bottom. I could feel her stretch and kick, and I blame her for the tenderness in my ribs. I could put my hand on top of my belly and feel her little bottom sticking up, while cupping my hand over my lower abdomen and feel her brother's head. Nothing can explain what it feels like to have two small babies moving inside your body, whether they are moving in sync or as the two separate beings that they are. I remember feeling Baby B bounce with hiccups, and in correspondence to her hiccups, Baby A would kick out. It was such a wild thought that they were interacting in this small way, reacting to each other's movements, and it was such a beautiful distraction from my discomfort.

And discomfort feels like a nice way of putting what I felt for most of my pregnancy. My pre-pregnancy jeans would no longer button as of the tenth week of pregnancy and the added weight affected my joints and muscles in ways I can barely even describe. However, my despair at not being able to fit into non-maternity jeans was completely overshadowed by the despair I felt when I reached the point of my pregnancy where I couldn't fit into *maternity* jeans. That's right. I couldn't wear clothing that was specifically made for pregnant women because I was simply too big. Don't be dismayed if you have to result to XXL men's shirts from Target, and don't feel pressured to wear pants. Attempting to wear pants while heavily pregnant with twins is almost physically impossible without enlisting the help of a handmaid. This is most certainly one of the main reasons we implemented a "call before coming over" policy. Because pants are overrated.

During the first portion of my pregnancy, I was struck with morning sickness that lasted all day long, which is common with twins due to the increase in your hormone levels. Whole days were spent on the couch as I battled nausea and tried to find a food that would benefit my babies and be easy on my stomach. My toddler learned to love television around this time because it was pretty much the only way I could survive the day-by-day trials of the first trimester, *que the mom-guilt*. By the time the morning sickness finally started to subside, I was already beginning to experience a lot of physical discomfort thanks to my increased size and weight load. There was so much extra weight from two babies, two placentas, and twice as much amniotic fluid that I felt so weighed down.

If you've ever been pregnant before, imagine what you felt at 40 weeks pregnant. That heavy, ready-to-burst, waddle-when-you-walk feeling of simply being full to capacity with the life inside you. That feeling started for me somewhere around week twenty-five. Walking was tiring and something that I tried to do in moderation. Too much of it made my back scream in protest, while the ligaments in my lower abdomen would ache from the strain of supporting my uterus. I couldn't stand for long periods of time without pretty much every part of my body aching. My legs and feet became swollen somewhere around twenty-six weeks into my pregnancy and didn't return to their normal size and shape until about six weeks postpartum. Sitting brought some relief, but it also caused my belly to push into my sternum, which hindered my breathing and gave me the kind of heartburn that radiated throughout my whole body. Did you know you could feel heartburn in your nostrils? Me either.

As my babies and I continued to grow, it became harder and harder to lug my body around. I literally felt as if a bowling ball was sitting in my pelvis and my movements felt sloth-like as I crawled through daily life. By the end of my pregnancy, my pubic bone was in such a constant state of pain that I remain fairly certain that it had fractured, which apparently is a thing that can happen. The more you know.

Fatigue was also a fairly abiding companion as my body was working overtime expending extra nutrients and calories to keep up with the rapid growth of the three of us inhabiting my 5'6" frame. My routine revolved around eating and sleeping, and there wasn't much energy left over for anything else. As if all this wasn't attractive enough, I also came to the conclusion that there wasn't so much a glow about me, as there was just a sheen of sweat from my forehead to my toes because I was incredibly hot all the time. I would say the blame for that fell partly on a twin pregnancy and partly on the fact that I was pregnant with twins in the summer in Texas. One hundred plus degrees Fahrenheit was not an ideal time to be carrying two humans and our electric bill reflected this. If you find yourself in a similar situation, I highly recommend the use of pools and cold showers (with a shower bench *obviously*). Pro tip: Sonic ice can be bought by the pound and is an ideal way to cool off while soothing said heartburn. You're welcome.

This was such a drastic deviation from my first pregnancy, and I had to really focus emotionally on making peace with this brand-new set of circumstances. It took me a long time to realize that growing two babies was going to be the pinnacle of my accomplishments over the nine-month duration of my pregnancy. Everything else on my to-do list was going to be resourced out while I watched and dictated from the couch. What your body needs at this time is rest, and so much of it while it performs the hard task that is growing two humans.

Despite the hardships, I was in complete awe of my body. I may have been freaking out slightly at the road ahead, but my body knew exactly what to do. It grew. It expanded. Day in and day out it worked gloriously to give my babies everything they needed. I walked away from my pregnancy with an entirely newfound appreciation for my body. When rest is what my body required of me, I rested. When it craved pancakes and strawberries, I went easy on the syrup and ate all of the strawberries. When my body was heavy and hard to carry, I sat and read twin birth stories and visualized how I wanted our pregnancy, labor, and delivery to go. It was a time for reflection, making healthy choices, and embracing the curveballs that came in life.

While I didn't have the energy to do much around the house, the down time gave me plenty of time to mediate, journal, and make a pretty considerable dent in my Netflix watch list. I also had plenty of time to snuggle my toddler. We would nap together every day, and I treasured those quiet moments of just the two of us knowing that it would soon end. It was forced relaxation, and during that time I made lists to keep up with everything I wanted and needed to get done before my babies arrived.

This downtime also let me see clearly the amazing people I have in my life. My husband, who has always been an incredible partner, truly made my pregnancy as relaxing as it could be. He cooked dinner every night and took our toddler to the grocery store on the weekends so I could rest. He offered to rub my legs when they would get sore after having muscle spasms all night long and picked up so much extra slack around the house that I simply couldn't get to. Nothing is sexier than seeing a man that works all day come home and fold clothes while making dinner and wearing a toddler on his back. If you want to highlight that last part for your partner to read, you have my permission.

My parents came to visit often and helped entertain our son and did small things around the house to help prepare for our twins. They folded onesies and hung curtains and offered me so much emotional support with their presence. My in-laws came and helped us set up the nursery so I wouldn't have to worry about it. They took care of our toddler, made dinner and ensured that we had everything we needed. When my son and I would venture to the park, my girlfriends would chase my son all over the playground so I wouldn't have to. Friends were constantly calling, texting, and asking what we needed as we got further and further along.

It was humbling and beautiful to see the love that surrounded us, and I may not have noticed it had I not been in a place where I couldn't do it all myself. It was frustrating not being able to physically tackle everything I wanted to, but to see our family and friends coming to our aid made my heart so full.

As you grow, waddle, and expend every ounce of strength and energy you have just making it to the bathroom in time, know that there will come a day when you will miss having your twins inside of your body. You will miss the swell of your belly, and the kicks into your ribs, bladder, and spine. As much as possible, which is sometimes so very hard, try to enjoy this time of growth for the beauty that it is. Find your silver linings and that spot of sweet warm sunshine that will carry you through the hard days and hold tight to them when the rain comes. You are doing something incredible during this time and it will pass quickly, despite how it may feel while you are in the thick of it. Once your babies are Earth side, it is a whole other ball game.

Chapter 3

Eating for Three

"Let food be thy medicine, and medicine be thy food."

Hippocrates

Of all the advice I've given over the last couple of years regarding twin pregnancy, my advice on nutrition is one I personally find to be the most vital to your overall pregnancy. The holistic approach to health is one that looks at nutrition as our first and primary defense against disease. It is one of the first subjects to be discussed and evaluated when considering wellness and prevention, as well as the primary culprit in many ills that plague the body.

What we put into our bodies for nourishment is so incredibly important to our overall health, and this is especially true when it comes to twin pregnancy. It only makes sense that nutrition plays such a huge role when life is being created. Your body is doing some of the hardest work it's ever done. You may not be running marathons, or physically tolling hours on end, but you are creating life. Two lives. Do not doubt for one second how incredibly hard your body is working, even if externally you can barely lift yourself from the couch.

In pregnancy, your body is not only creating your babies, but it is creating a new organ specifically for your babies called the placenta. If you are having Di/Di twins, then your body is creating two placentas. Your blood volume level increases during pregnancy to support your growing baby by about 45%, and the increase is even more so in a twin pregnancy at almost 60%. This increase in blood volume is all part of your body's grand design to provide your babies with the nutrients it needs. The excess blood flow helps transport vitamins, nutrients, and hormones to the placenta.

The placenta is connected to your uterine wall and its main function is to extract nutrients from your body to give to your babies via the umbilical cord. The more babies in your uterus, the greater the nutrient drain on your body. This is why nutrition in pregnancy is vital to your health and the health of your babies. The nutrients you provide your body with will go on to be the nutrients that your babies receive, and the more nutrients your babies receive, the better and healthier they grow and develop. You have to give your body the best in order for your babies to receive the best. You also have to be mindful of your own nutritional needs to support your growing body as best as you can. Going forward, it is in you and your babies' best interest to view food as the life source that it is. Everything you eat should be bringing you closer to your daily caloric and nutritional goals.

For a twin pregnancy, your goal should be to add 600 extra calories a day to your diet; 300 extra calories for each baby. That being said, I think it is important to not get too hung up on calorie count or weight gain. You are not a cow being fattened for slaughter. You are a goddess trying to provide the best nutrition possible for your babies. Don't feel pressured to eat every hour, or to eat when you aren't hungry, or meet an unrealistic goal of "xyz" calories. More than anything, your focus should be on eating a balanced, healthy diet on a timeline and schedule that feels good to you.

Protein:

Protein during pregnancy will be one of the most important things you can give your body. Protein is a macronutrient that is composed of amino acids. Its primary function within our bodies is to help regulate the function and regeneration of cells, tissues, and organs. It helps your body with uterine tissue support and is responsible for increasing your blood supply. It is vital for helping your baby develop their brain and fetal tissue.

Recent studies have found that mothers of multiples who focused on a nutrient dense, high protein diet throughout the duration of pregnancy had a tendency to carry their babies closer to term, with improved birth weights of the babies. Dr. William Goodnight and Dr. Roger Newman published a study specifically relating to multiples pregnancy and the impact of nutrition. Their conclusion was that there is a correlation between maternal diet and gestation duration, and that nutrition should be a primary focus when carrying multiples. Their study builds on the existing theory by Dr. Thomas Brewer that protein intake plays a vital role in helping a mother of multiples meet the increased nutritional demands that come with a multiples pregnancy. Dr. Brewer consistently found that mothers who take greater care in meeting these nutritional demands tend to have less complications associated with a multiples pregnancy, and longer gestations, than those who don't. Dr. Brewer's recommendation, based on decades of research and hands-on studies, indicate a need for at least 120-150 grams of protein daily.

If you are a meat eater, you will find the bulk of your protein in beef, poultry, and pork. Fish, eggs, milk and cheese are also good sources of animal-based protein. Protein from animals is considered to be a complete protein as it has all nine components of the essential amino acids that your body needs and can't produce on its own. However, many women choose to avoid meat and animal-based products for personal, religious, or health reasons. Being pregnant doesn't automatically mean that you need to revamp your diet, as long as you are daily striving to provide your body with a variety of foods that have a high range of nutritional value. Meat offers an easy solution to meeting your protein demands, but it is possible to consume the protein you need while avoiding it. Some plant-based sources of protein tend to be deficient of certain amino acids making it an "incomplete" source of protein; however, buckwheat, quinoa, soy, and hemp seeds are considered to have all nine of the amino acids and should be a staple in any meatless diet.

In addition to high quality proteins, Dr. Brewer recommended that your diet include a variety of fresh fruits and vegetables, unrefined whole grains, healthy fats and oils, and foods rich in vitamin A and C. The best way to get the most out of the food you eat is to incorporate a real and whole foods approach that places an emphasis on the quality and freshness of your food.

A whole foods diet means that your food is as unrefined and unprocessed as possible. Fresh fruit and vegetables, high quality meats, and meals that are made with organic and fresh ingredients will go so much further in aiding your nutritional demands than, say, a fast food burger. In pregnancy, you also need calcium, folate acid, iron, and a variety of vitamins to truly meet your nutritional needs and those of your babies.

Calcium:

Calcium is essential in strengthening and developing your baby's bones. While it's obvious that dairy is one of the highest sources of calcium (milk, cheese, yogurt, and cottage cheese are great sources of calcium from dairy), it is possible to receive calcium from plant sources.

Seeds like poppy, sesame, and chia are especially rich in calcium. Lentils, beans, dark leafy greens like kale, spinach, and collard greens, almonds, edamame, and dried figs are all great non-dairy sources of calcium. The bonus is that most of the plant-based calcium sources are also rich in other needed nutrients like fiber, folate, magnesium, healthy fats, copper, iron, and protein.

Folate Acid:

Folate acid is a form of Vitamin B9. Studies have shown that a maternal diet high in folate acid reduces risks of birth defects like spina bifida (spinal deficiency) and anencephaly (brain growth anomaly), as folate acid helps with the generation of brain tissue. Folate acid is essential to helping cells form, divide, and regenerate as well as making and repairing DNA. It's easy to see why this is such an important nutrient to have in pregnancy. Folate acid is only found in food as it is the natural occurring source of vitamin B9. Folic acid is the synthetic version of vitamin B9. Many people consider folate and folic acid to be interchangeable due to the fact that their molecular structure is nearly identical; however, the way your body process each is different. Folate, the naturally occurring form, is converted to active vitamin B9 while in your stomach as it's being digested. Folic does not convert to active vitamin B9 until it reaches your liver. As a result, folic acid does not get metabolized in your system until much later. This can cause folic acid to build up in your system with adverse health effects. The best way to ensure that you are getting the best benefit of vitamin B9 is by absorbing folate through your diet. Folate acid can be found in dark leafy greens like spinach, kale, and arugula, as well as asparagus, Brussel sprouts, avocados, legumes (beans and lentils), eggs, flaxseeds, broccoli, and bananas.

Iron:

Iron is important for creating and sustaining blood cells that your body uses to transport vital nutrients throughout your body and into the placenta. It also aids in delivering oxygen to your babies. Your body uses iron to help make the 60% extra blood that your body needs during pregnancy as well.

Iron is broken down into two forms: heme and nonheme. Heme iron is found in blood and muscles and as such, can only be gotten through a meat diet (beef, pork, poultry, and turkey). Nonheme iron is found in things like legumes (lentils, chickpeas, lima and kidney beans, soybeans, tofu, and tempeh), quinoa, nuts and seeds (hemp, flaxseed, cashews, pine nuts, pumpkin and sesame), leafy greens (spinach, kale, collard greens, and swiss chard), potato skins, and mushrooms. Iron that is gleaned from plant-based sources are not absorbed into your body as easily as the iron that you receive from meat, but there are ways to help your body with absorption. Studies suggest that pairing your iron intake with Vitamin C or lysine-rich foods (quinoa, legumes, bell peppers) can help your body absorb it better. Things like coffee and tea are found to hinder iron absorption, so it is recommended to avoid these beverages while your body is digesting iron rich foods. Cooking with a cast iron pan is also a great way to get a bit of extra iron in your diet. Last but not least, iron can also be found in dark chocolate, so do with that information what you will.

While your doctor or midwife will more than likely recommend a prenatal supplement to help you receive these nutrients, it is important that you strive to get as much as you can from your food intake. Vitamin supplements are not intended to replace a healthy diet. Whatever your babies do not receive from your diet, they will take from your own body's reserves. Over time, this can cause you, the mother and life source, to have a deficiency. As with all things, you need to listen to your body and make the best and healthiest decisions for yourself.

The Science:

Dr. Brewer first began studying the correlation between maternal diet and healthy birth rates in 1950 when he was attempting to discover why some women fell victim to disease in pregnancy. His studies found that when women did not eat enough protein, or enough protein coupled with adequate calories, her body responded by going into preservation mode. The goal of this preservation was not necessarily preservation of self, but rather preservation of the baby at all costs, even to the detriment of the mother.

The liver is responsible for making albumin which helps increase the blood volume, but Dr. Brewer found that the liver can only make albumin with the protein from the mother's diet. When protein and adequate calories are absent from a mother's diet, the liver does not make albumin and the blood volume begins to suffer. The kidneys automatically respond to this dip in blood volume by producing an enzyme called renin which makes the blood vessels constrict. This in itself is an act of preservation due to the fact that a sudden drop in blood volume signals to your kidneys that you are more than likely hemorrhaging. Your kidney's response to this perceived hemorrhage is to try to mitigate damage by reducing blood flow to your hands, feet, and organs. When you are not hemorrhaging, but rather simply not meeting your body's nutritional demands, this restriction of blood vessels causes the blood pressure to rise. At this point, your kidneys cannot increase the blood volume though it keeps trying by reabsorbing the fluid that it has already filtered. As a result, the blood that it keeps trying to reabsorb gets leaked into your tissues causing swelling and rapid weight gain. This creates what the medical community recognizes as preeclampsia.

In the 1950's, when women were still sanctioned to safely smoke cigarettes and drink alcohol during pregnancy, this was a huge breakthrough in the way we viewed a mother's overall health and its impact on pregnancy. Upon discovering this link between diet and disease, Dr. Brewer's passion was born, and his research grew into the highly respected work that it is today. Thanks to his dedication and research, he was able to link maternal diet to a variety of issues that plagued pregnant women such as toxemia, placental abruption, pre-eclampsia and pre-term labor. His work was groundbreaking, but the idea that nutrition is so vital to pregnancy is still considered to be somewhat in the realm of "alternative" medicine, and thus is treated as such. Even today, almost 70 years later, most obstetricians do not place the proper emphasis on the importance of a healthy diet to expecting mothers.

I recently conducted a poll of mothers who are pregnant with twins and was shocked to discover that 72% of them were not educated on the importance of nutrition and/or protein in their diets by their obstetricians, and a further 20% of them were told that nutrition plays no role in the health of their babies or the length of gestation. The fact that nutrition is downplayed among obstetricians is disheartening, especially in light of Dr. Brewer, Dr. Goodnight, and Dr. Newman's findings that clearly link the two. There are many nutrition experts and scientific studies that are now realizing the importance that diet plays in the role of prevention of disease and common pregnancy ailments; however, this information is not being consistently made available to the women who need it.

Heidi Murkoff, author of What to Expect When Expecting, has started following in Dr. Brewer's footsteps with her Pregnancy Diet Plan also putting a heavy emphasis on protein intake during pregnancy, with the recommendation being on 100 grams of protein daily. Her research, coupled with research done through the Centers for Disease Control, National Institute of Health, the Food and Drug Administration, and the American College of Obstetrics and Gynecologists have confirmed Dr. Brewer's findings that a proper maternal diet can be instrumental in helping prevent preeclampsia, gestational diabetes, and preterm labor, as well as supporting placental integrity (including abruption prevention and efficiency into later pregnancy).

We are at a delicate point in time where the science supporting the impact of nutrition is there, but the practice, application and education of it within the medical community is lagging behind. Do not be afraid to address nutrition with your doctor or midwife to find out their views on the importance of it in regard to your pregnancy.

It is vital, more now than ever, that you as a woman and mother do your own research and advocate for your health and the health of your babies. I know it can seem daunting to look at the nutrition your body needs (especially if you are still struggling with nausea, and then later, struggling with room in your stomach for more than a few bites) but your nutrition is one of the most important things you can take control of within your twin pregnancy. Eating the right foods to support your body and your babies is now your obligation. Grazing throughout the day on small but protein and nutrient packed snacks is one way to help you meet your goal. An app, like MyFitnessPal, can be used to help you keep track of what you eat so that you are consistently meeting your nutritional goals. I truly believe that a healthy diet with a focal point on protein intake and fresh vegetables can make a huge difference in the outcome of your twin pregnancy.

Hydration:

Another very important element to your diet, both now and always, is water. Water is essential to every living thing, and again, even more so when creating life. Due to an increase in hormones, women have a tendency to sweat more in pregnancy, and the added weight from your growing babies also increases your core temperature and leads to an increase of water being evaporated from your skin. You are also probably urinating more frequently due to your bladder being kicked around, but also due in part to the fact that your kidneys are actually producing more urine by about 25% thanks to the 60% increased blood flow. Sweating, evaporation, and urination all lead to hydration loss and it is vital to replenish that water loss. I cannot stress it enough, hydrate, hydrate, hydrate. Aside from meeting your nutritional goals, it is one of the best things you can give your body at this time.

I know what you're thinking; more water means more peeing, and when you are already making more trips to the bathroom than feels humanly possible it can be seem like a dismaying venture. However, it is worth it. A healthy you and healthy babies makes it all worth it.

The Science:

The National Academies Health and Medicine Division (formerly known as The Institute of Medicine) recommends that pregnant women drink 3 liters, or roughly 100 ounces, of water a day.

While pregnant, I consumed just over the recommendation at 3.7 liters, or 128 ounces (a gallon). It was an amount that both my midwife and I felt comfortable with. It is important to listen to your body and set a realistic goal that feels right for you. Feeling thirsty is a sign that you are already lacking in adequate hydration. The color of your urine will also tell you a lot about how hydrated your body is; however, keep in mind that some vitamins and supplements can change the color of your urine output so this may not be a reliable way to judge whether or not you are dehydrated. Urine should be pale yellow in color. Urine that is clear means you are drinking too much water, or possibly drinking it too quickly, and urine that is bright yellow means you are certainly not getting enough.

As previously mentioned, your body is sending nutrients to your babies via the placenta, and it does so with the help of water. In day to day life, water is responsible for delivering oxygen and nutrients to our skin, organs, and cells so that our bodies are continually regenerating. In pregnancy, the water helps transport these nutrient rich blood cells right to your babies through the placenta.

Experts believe that water intake in pregnancy also helps your baby's amniotic fluid regenerate. The more water you drink, the better equipped your placenta is to continue giving your baby the nutrients it needs and keep the protective fluid at just the right levels. Amniotic fluid is vital to your baby's development in many ways. In utero, babies practice both breathing and drinking by swallowing the amniotic fluid. It helps their kidneys begin functioning even as they continue to develop, as well as their bladders as they urinate the fluid back out into their sacs. Adequate hydration from you will ensure that the amniotic fluid properly renews as needed so your babies can continue growing and developing inside and out.

Proper water intake and hydration, while essential for your baby's growth and development, isn't just for your baby's benefit. When you are well hydrated, you will find that you are much more comfortable. Proper water intake can help flush your body of toxins and excess sodium which reduces issues with edema (swelling of hands, feet, and legs). While swelling is typically not painful, it can be bothersome and uncomfortable.

Adequate water intake also aids in the absorption of vital nutrients and helps your digestive tract function properly to prevent constipation, which can occur due to restricted room in your lower abdomen and hormonal changes that tend to slow down your digestion. Constipation in turn can lead to feeling even more uncomfortable and can cause hemorrhoids due to straining to relieve yourself. Water consumption helps your body break down waste better so that it can pass more easily through your system. Water can also help reduce the chances of developing urinary tract infections both in the bladder and the kidneys, which is a common problem in pregnancy due to your growing uterus pressing into your bladder and hindering you from being able to properly and completely empty your bladder as needed. Without being able to properly empty your bladder, urine can back up into the kidneys and cause pain, inflammation, and infections. Kidney pain is never fun, and it is even less so when you are already struggling with the comforts, or lack therefore, in a twin pregnancy.

Keeping hydrated is especially important in the later stages of pregnancy, as dehydration can cause contractions and even lead to preterm labor, as well as cause drastic blood pressure changes. If a sudden change occurs in your blood pressure, you risk fainting or dizziness. Dehydration is also responsible for headaches and fatigue, both of which you might possibly also have in spades due to the pregnancy hormones.

Water is also a good way to stay cool, even as your body temperature rises a bit. Between your body constantly working to create your babies, the hormones, and your overall added weight to your body, overheating can happen easily and the best way to keep your core cool is to stay hydrated throughout the day.

If drinking a lot of water is not something you are in the habit of doing, it might help to carry a water bottle with you at all times. Fill a gallon pitcher of water every morning and make it your goal to finish it by the time night rolls around. If water is not something you enjoy to drink, or even like to drink, think about adding fruits or vegetables to it. Lemons, limes, and cucumbers are a nice addition to a cold glass of water. Coconut water is a tasty supplement as well, and it is full of electrolytes. Electrolytes are sodium that our bodies use to help regulate the flow of water in and out of our cells.

Find something that works for you and do your best to make hydration a priority throughout your pregnancy. Again, it is important to listen to your body and do what feels right and good for you. Do not stress to drink a gallon of water a day if it simply does not feel good. I truly believe that if you listen to your body and follow your instincts you can't go wrong. Moderation is key.

What you eat and drink throughout your pregnancy matters greatly. At a time when there are a lot of unknowns and various factors that you can't always control, diet is one of the things you can take into your hands. It is up to you to ensure that you are giving your body and your babies the best every single day. Eat up, drink up, and know that every nutrient loaded morsel you eat will be put to good use.

Chapter 4

Finding your Tribe

"It takes a village to raise a child, but it takes a tribe to raise a mother."

Unknown

We've talked about science, placentas, discomfort, and the importance of quality food and water intake, so now let's talk about doctors and midwives. One of the first things on your to-do list after finding out you are pregnant should be finding a good provider. Prenatal care is incredibly important, as is building up a support system around you as you continue through your pregnancy. Your medical provider can be an excellent source of support as long as they are chosen with care. Whom you choose to support and surround you during pregnancy will have an impact not only on your pregnancy, but on your labor and birth as well.

Knowing What you Want:

Before delving into the ins-and-outs of finding a medical provider, however, it is essential to determine exactly what type of birth you want. What do you want out of your birth experience? Do you want an epidural? Do you want a medication-free delivery? Do you want to birth in a hospital? A birth center? At home? In the sea with dolphins? (I'm just joking with the last one. Please do not attempt to birth in the ocean.) Have you even thought that far ahead?

Now is the time to start thinking about and preparing for the birth that you desire. If you are a new mother, birth can seem mysterious and scary. It may be something that you've had no real-life experience with at all, and the prospect of giving birth to two humans can seem daunting. However, I believe that birth is what you make it. It can be a beautiful, empowering experience if that is what you desire, and as a woman creating life you can have a say in what happens.

At times, the options that a mother has regarding birth are not always obvious or even talked about, due largely in part to the fact that some of the options are not considered mainstream. When it comes to twin pregnancy and delivery, it seems as if there are even fewer discussions of your options.

Until my pregnancy with my first child, I assumed there was only one way to birth a baby. Go to the hospital, get poked, prodded and possibly cut open, have a baby and go home. It wasn't until I started doing research into birthing options that I realized there was more than one way to go about it. The type of birth you want will be determined by the care you seek. There are some countries in the world where midwives work hand-in-hand with obstetricians and are employed through hospitals; however, in the United States midwives and their practices are typically independent of hospital affiliations. This means that in the US there are three main options regarding birth: seeking out an OBGYN and delivering in a hospital or finding a midwife and delivering either at home or in a stand-alone birth center that operates independently of a hospital. By determining what you want your birth to look like, you will have a better idea of the type of care you will need and the type of provider to look for.

Your medical provider is an essential part of your prenatal care, and not just any provider will do. As with any relationship you build in life, there needs to be a solid foundation of respect and trust between you and your care provider. You are, in essence, placing your life and the lives of your children into this person's hands. It is vital that you find someone that you can openly communicate with. Someone who you intrinsically trust, and someone who values you as a woman and respects your insight, intuition, and wishes. This may take some doing. You may need to visit with many doctors or midwives before finding someone that is right for you. Ask questions and press hard for answers. Know what their comforts and limitations are when it comes to caring for a multiples pregnancy and what their experience with twin delivery is. I cannot overstate this enough: it is so important that you feel valued and safe with your care provider.

My first obstetrician received many positive reviews on her website. Many women loved her and had nothing but wonderful things to say about her. However, after a few visits, I quickly realized that we were not a good fit. Many of my desires for birth did not align with her practices. I was hoping for a medication free birth, with no interventions. She did not have faith that I could achieve it, nor was she willing to let my body naturally go into labor as I desired. My pregnancy, in her eyes, had an expiration date of her choosing. I went back to square one and began researching medical providers who would be more supportive of my desires.

It was at this time that I discovered midwifery. I instantly felt that it was a wonderful fit for me, much more so than the standard model of care you find within traditional obstetrics. The midwife model of care is family centered and includes attending to both the physical and emotional well-being of the mother from conception to postpartum. It tends to lean more to holistic and natural care, with as little intervention as possible with the focus being on whole food nutrition, natural supplements, and empowerment on behalf of the mother to know and trust her body and baby. Care plans tend to be individualized to each woman, with regard to meeting her emotional, mental, and physical needs.

Knowing now what I wanted, I set about finding the right midwife for me. The provider that I connected with and felt comfortable with. For this huge journey of bringing children into the world, I wanted someone that I instantly had a rapport with. Someone who looked at me as a person and respected my wishes. I stumbled onto a beautiful birth center just ten miles from our home, and upon meeting with the owner and midwife Kim Daly, I knew I had found my medical provider. She patiently guided me through a tour of the facilities, explaining how they operated and then took over an hour to answer every single question I had, which says a lot considering I had over three pages of questions. She was warm and personable, open and inviting, and she reinforced my desires for my birth. From day one, I knew that she truly wanted the best for me and my babies. She believed in me and encouraged me to believe in myself. She was an excellent source of support and informational resources, and I truly believe she helped make my pregnancy as successful as it could be. She was reassuring when I needed it. She was calm when I was stressed. She was encouraging at every step and stage when I began to doubt myself. She provided a wealth of insight and information that proved invaluable to this whole process, and I could not have done it without her. My pregnancy and births were everything I wanted because I sought out the right person to support me.

I know not everyone wants to labor medication free, and I completely support that. This chapter is not about pushing the midwife agenda on anyone that desperately wants an epidural, it is about making sure you know your options, your desires are respected, and your plans are supported. As a woman, I want to you to feel empowered by the birthing process, whatever that looks like to you, and a huge part of that is being on the same page as your care provider. Birth can be a beautiful, transformative experience if that is what you desire. There tends to be a culture of fear surrounding what has come to be seen as an unpredictable and scary experience, and you don't have to look hard to find horror stories surrounding birth. However, I like to think that these stories are the exception and not the rule. That birth can be an empowering and amazing experience. I think a large part of that is what you walk into birth with; your expectations, your desires, your willingness to fight for what it will be for you.

The most important thing at this stage is to learn to be an advocate for yourself and your babies. Know what you want and strive to find someone who will respect you and your wishes. You are not another number, or a statistic. You are a woman bringing life into this world. It is an incredible and amazing time of your life and every person you allow into your inner circle should be in absolute awe of that.

Ask around, inquire with your local Moms of Multiples group, do your homework. Don't be afraid to shop doctors or midwives until you find someone you can trust and feel safe with, who will treat you with the respect that you as a person deserve. It is never too late to change providers if you feel that you are not receiving the support or care you deserve. Do not be afraid to change course during your pregnancy if the need arises. This is your pregnancy and your body, and you are entitled to find a provider that will strive to meet your needs. Having a great relationship with your care provider makes it easier to trust them during labor in the event that something unexpected happens and birth plans need to be adjusted.

Midwifery vs Traditional Obstetrics: Legalities:

There are pros and cons to both models of care. If you choose to birth at home or a birth center, there might be red tape involved. In the United States, midwifery laws vary from state to state. Some states allow twins to be born at home or in a stand-alone birth center (a birthing center that is completely separate from a hospital and is run by midwives), while some states do not allow twin births to occur outside of a hospital setting. It is important to do a little research and learn what feasibly can and cannot be done within your state (or country).

Another con to attempting to have your baby outside of the hospital is the possibility that something changes last minute, or during labor, (i.e. a baby becomes distressed, or labor does not progress as needed) and you will have to transfer to a hospital. This means you would incur more cost in the long run as you will have to pay for both your midwife and the hospital stay. In this particular scenario, it also means that you will be delivering with a doctor you do not know or have any sort of rapport with.

Another con to an out of hospital delivery is in the event of a true emergency, you are not in a hospital. Most midwives are diligent in their care and strive to ensure that true emergencies are rare. Most of the time, complications can be found in a timely enough fashion that it is dealt with before becoming a true emergency. In this situation, I am defining a true emergency as something that could be potentially life threatening to either mother or babies. This is why most midwives take the proper steps to ensure that the pregnancy progresses with as few complications as possible. An uncomplicated pregnancy tends to continue on with an uncomplicated labor and delivery.

With the standard route of obstetrics and hospital births, you can expect to find a few cons as well. Many hospitals and doctors will urge you to be induced by 37 weeks in a standard Mo/Di pregnancy, by 38 weeks in a standard Di/Di pregnancy, and between 32-34 weeks in a standard Mo/Mo pregnancy. The idea behind this is usually fear based: doctors fear that the placenta may begin to deteriorate the longer a twin pregnancy runs. However, as we covered in chapter three, I believe good nutrition goes a long way to ensuring that your body and placenta continue operating the way it was designed to.

I personally believe that babies come when babies are ready, and any time before that is interfering with the natural process. While the last few weeks of any pregnancy can feel like a waiting game, especially when you are full term with twins, your body is still continuing to do hard work even up to the 11th hour. Intricacies of your baby's brain and lungs are still being formed up until 40 weeks gestation. Allowing your body to carry your babies as long as possible ensures that their bodies are formed perfectly. Induction, while it is an intervention with the body's natural process, is not necessarily a con within itself, though some believe that inducing a woman to go into labor before her body or babies are ready increases the likely hood of a caesarean.

The Cascade of Interventions is a term that refers to the idea that once an intervention has been introduced to the process it creates a new problem that requires a new intervention, and thus the cycle goes. In terms of childbirth, an induction increases the likelihood of an epidural which increases the likelihood of a caesarean. With an induction, the body is receiving synthetic hormones to jump-start the labor process. This can cause the process to do one of two things: stall with failure to progress, or it can cause such strong contractions that there is an increased need for medication. Having an epidural restricts your movement and ability to naturally work through contractions and settle into positions that are known to help bring your baby down into the birth canal which in turn can cause fetal distress. Once fetal distress is detected, you are well on your way to a C-section.

Another con to delivering via the standard route is that most hospitals in the United States requires that a twin birth take place within the

Operating Room regardless of whether or not you plan for their births to be vaginal. It is an administrative move that mitigates risks, and a lot of times it is out of a doctor's hands. If you have been in an operating room before then you know that these spaces are brightly lit, stark, and cold. This may not bother some women, but studies have shown that these things tend to hinder the birthing process. A softly lit, warm space is more conducive to the birthing process and allows a woman to birth more comfortably. When a woman feels safe and secure in her surroundings, birth tends to progress more easily.

Armed with this information, it is in your hands to make the best choice for you and your babies. You have to advocate for yourself and take your health into your own hands. I feel fortunate that I live in a state that allows twin births to occur outside of the hospital, and that I had an amazing midwife willing to help me achieve my desire for a natural, intervention-free birth. I felt supported and respected throughout every step of my pregnancy, and that is my wish for every woman, no matter how or where she chooses to birth.

Chapter 5

Caesarean Vs. Vaginal

"There is a secret in our culture, and it's not that birth is painful. It's that women are strong."

Laura Stavoe Harm

When it comes to having a twin pregnancy, you are hard pressed to find a story that does not end with a cesarean. This is due mainly in part to the fact that in the United States a 2008 study showed that 75% of all twin pregnancies end in C-section, despite the fact that there is no evidence that it is safer to either babies or mother, nor is it particularly warranted simply because there are two babies in the womb. Wikipedia lists twin pregnancy as a reason for women to undergo a C-section, so please let me repeat: having two babies growing inside your body is not reason enough to undergo a caesarean.

Despite overwhelming evidence that vaginal birth is a safe option for twin delivery, many doctors do not feel comfortable allowing a twin birth to play out naturally simply because it hasn't been seen as the traditional option. Many doctors and residents go their entire careers without ever seeing what a vaginal twin birth looks like up close and personal. There is no hands-on experience that allows them to see how beautifully a twin delivery can be managed. Therefore, when having to choose between an unknown vaginal delivery with twins, and a caesarean, many doctors decide to go a route they know and are more comfortable with.

I believe there is a time and place for caesarean births. It is at times a necessary option that can save lives, and it takes an incredibly strong woman to embrace this route for the sake of giving life to her children. It is not an easy out, nor does it diminish the act of giving birth. Woman are strong and amazing no matter how their babies come into the world. My desire for a natural birth was born out of my intense fear of needles and hospitals. I do not find natural birth to be a superior option, it was simply the ideal option for me. I look at women who have undergone cesareans as superheroes. Not only have they had a major surgery for the sake of their child, but they then go on to care for this new human while in recovery and I believe there is truly no greater love than this. I realize that there are times and situations beyond our control that call for surgical intervention. I realize that this is a reality for many women, whether they are pregnant with twins or not, and I recognize the importance and value that cesareans can have in moments of emergency. However, in recent years, and especially in regard to twin pregnancy, cesareans have become less about necessity and true emergency intervention, and more about convenience and comfort on the part of the doctor.

A cesarean section, for those who do not know the specifics, is a surgical procedure that removes the baby directly from the uterus. A woman is either given a spinal block to numb her so that she is awake but cannot feel the pain of the procedure, or medication is pushed through a catheter port at the spine (epidural), or she is put under general anesthesia which means she is completely unconscious. Most medical professionals try to use a spinal block or epidural when they can, but in instances of an emergency C-section general anesthesia is often used. A cut is then made to her lower abdomen, and a second cut is made to her uterus. The babies and placenta(s) are pulled out, then the incisions are stitched closed.

Fetal Positioning:

In recent years, studies have shown that a C-section isn't always necessary in twin delivery and that vaginal birth can be a safe and viable option with the support of a knowledgeable attending doctor or midwife.

In most circumstances, but not all, the ease with which you can deliver your babies vaginally is dependent on their position within your uterus. Your babies will move all over the place throughout your pregnancy and their positions could be up, down, or sideways depending on the day. Their position does not become important until you progress through the third trimester, and most providers don't consider abnormal positioning to be worrisome until weeks 33 or later. At this stage of your baby's growth and development, their head begins to take on more weight than their body.

This increase in weight, combined with gravity, are what naturally pull your baby's head down toward the opening of your uterus. This head-down position, known as cephalic presentation or vertex, is the optimal position for vaginal birth, in both a singleton and twin delivery. In the vertex position, your baby is head-down against the opening of your uterus, with their chin tucked and their legs and arms tucked into their body. If your baby is facing your back, this is referred to as anterior, while a head-down baby facing out towards your belly button is considered posterior.

Breech babies are positioned with their head up towards your ribs. There are three variations of breech: Frank, complete, and Footling. Frank breech is where the baby has its butt toward the birth canal, with their feet towards their head. Complete breech is when their butt is toward the birth canal with their knees bent and feet down by their butt. Footling breech is when their butt is down and either one or both of their feet are hanging down toward the birth canal. There is a small risk of complications with breech vaginal birth, as the baby's head is the last thing to leave the mother's body. There is an increased risk that your baby can get stuck in the birth canal or lose oxygen as the cord can get compressed between the head and the canal; however, this risk remains quite small and many healthy babies have been delivered breech.

The last position, and most uncommon, is transverse. In a transverse position your baby is horizontally across your belly, and vaginal birth is considered dangerous to attempt due to the increased risk of complications. Many babies that are transverse in early pregnancy tend to rotate head down as you get nearer to your due date. At one point in my pregnancy, my twin b was lying transverse across the top of my belly, but within a week or two she rotated head down, so a transverse presentation is not something to worry about unless you are approaching the later weeks of pregnancy. Even then, it is still possible for your baby to rotate to the optimal position before labor begins unless space and ability to flip have become an issue.

As stated, vertex is the ideal and most common position for vaginal delivery as their head first presentation makes for an easier and smoother path through the vaginal canal; however, babies can be born breech. There are considered to be more risks associated with breech birth, and while the risks are minimal, some doctors and midwives refuse to assist or advocate for vaginal delivery if one or more of your babies are in the breech position. However, some midwives and doctors are more experienced with breech delivery than others and would be willing to attempt a vaginal birth in the event that one or both babies are breech, which is another reason that it is important to carefully choose your medical provider. A vertex/breech combination is fairly common with twin pregnancy, and it is important to know how comfortable your care provider is in allowing an attempted vaginal birth in this instance. Some providers are more comfortable with vaginal delivery in which Twin A is vertex and Twin B is breech due to the expectation that Twin A widens the birth canal enough that the second breech baby can progress through it more easily.

Statistics and Trial Studies: The Case for Vaginal:

A medical study done out of Ireland followed over four hundred women expecting twins and found no significant difference in the perinatal outcome of vaginal births than that with women who chose an elective C-section.

A 2015 study conducted by the Brigham and Women's Hospital in Boston, Massachusetts had similar findings with the results of the trial study urging obstetricians to consider vaginal delivery above C-sections when Twin A was presenting vertex. The Brigham and Women's Hospital is the second largest teaching affiliate (Harvard Medical School) and their studies are urging doctors across the United States to allow twin vaginal births to play out, with caesarean being a last resort to delivery.

Another study done by Maternite Port-Royal, in Paris, France did a similar study and found that 78.4% of women attempting to birth twins vaginally were successful, while 21.1% had a cesarean during labor, and only .5% ended up needing a Cesarean for twin B only. Their conclusion following the study found that planned vaginal delivery was a safe option for twins with a gestation age of 32 weeks or older that had Twin A presenting vertex.

A study done out of Walter Sisulu University in South Africa actually set out to prove that routine Cesareans for twin pregnancies was a safer alternative to eliminate the risks found in vaginal twin birth; however, their study conclusion was that there was no evidence to support planned caesarean's for twin pregnancies in which Twin A was vertex and that to continue performing C-sections with the sole intention of mitigating risks of vaginal birth was not a credible way to avoid risks.

These multiple studies done across multiple continents have all found the same thing: that vaginal birth is a safe, and at times an expected option, when the pregnancy has been fairly low risk, the babies have reached term, and Twin A is vertex.

I lay this information out to you so that you can know your options. So that you can feel confident in your choices and desires for your birth. There is too much misinformation regarding what birthing twins looks like, and unfortunately, that misinformation tends to leave women thinking that there is only one way forward when that is simply not the case. Growing two humans is an enormous and amazing task, but it doesn't automatically limit you in your options when it comes to bringing them into this world.

Note that a Mo/Mo pregnancy is at higher risk of birth complications than a Di/Di or Mo/Di pregnancy because of the shared sac and placenta. Many doctors and midwives refuse to consider vaginal delivery of Mo/Mo twins due to the increased risks that this type of pregnancy can entail. If you are carrying Mo/Mo twins it is important that you discuss your delivery options with your care provider.

Caesarean Risks:

While cesareans are needed in certain situations like placenta previa (when the placenta lies over the opening of the uterus), or transverse positioning, it does carry more risks than vaginal birth. The National Health Service in the United Kingdom estimated that the risk of maternal death during a C-section is three times that of a vaginal birth, due mainly in part to blood clots (a common postoperative complication), infections of the incision site, and complications associated with undergoing anesthesia.

A caesarean, while somewhat common (especially in the United States), is still a very serious medical procedure that has more risks associated with it than vaginal birth. Postpartum hemorrhage has been shown to be greater in caesarean sections than vaginal births, and some women have issues with wound hematoma, which is when the wound bleeds profusely and can't be stopped.

Women who have undergone a Caesarean incurs more risk in future births. Her choices when preparing to birth again are to either choose another caesarean or to attempt a vaginal birth. A vaginal birth that occurs after a caesarean is referred to as a VBAC (vaginal birth after caesarean). Both options present a higher set of risks. A vaginal birth that is attempted after a caesarean carries the risk of uterine rupture, endometriosis, and postpartum hemorrhage, while another caesarean increases risks of hemorrhage, blood clots, and an increase in abdominal scar tissue that can interfere with fertility, cause chronic pelvic pain, and lead to obstruction of the bowels. A second caesarean after a previous one also poses a risk for uterine rupture due to the scar tissue of the previous incision site weakening. If the uterus ruptures, it can quickly become life threatening for both mother and baby. Scar tissue can also cause placental problems in future pregnancies.

Babies born via caesarean are at greater risk of having breathing issues at birth. One theory is that a vaginal birth allows a baby's chest to compress as it goes through the birth canal which squeezes out excess fluid from the lungs. A baby born via caesarean does not have this advantage. Studies have also shown that babies born via caesarean carry an additional risk of developing asthma in childhood, as well as other infections and diseases due mainly in part to the fact that a Caesarean birth prevents the baby from benefitting from the good bacteria that is found within the mother's birth canal and vagina. Exposure to this good bacterium, often referred to as flora, is said to help boost the baby's immune system, and introduce a healthy microbiome to their stomach that helps with the prevention of disease both in the short- and long-term span of their lives.

While these risks can sound alarming, please know that these are the exception and not the rule. Many women safely have cesareans all over the world every day for a variety of reasons. It is important that you know what you are facing when weighing your options.

Vaginal Birth Risks:

There are, of course, risks associated with vaginal births as well. Tearing of the perineum (skin below the vagina) is a common one. Though most tears are minor requiring only a stitch or two, they can be severe with extensive stitching required. Tears of the perineum can be prevented if a mother is allowed to rest as baby's head draws near the vaginal opening. Some midwives and doctors will even coach a woman to slow down and breathe through the last phase of pushing in an attempt to let the body naturally stretch to reduce risk of tears. The pelvic floor can become damaged or weakened during the pushing phase as well, causing a woman to experience bowel issues or incontinence if untreated. After a vaginal birth, a woman may experience lingering pain in the skin and tissue surrounding the vagina. Most women recover within 6 weeks of childbirth. However, if a birth was especially hard or extensive pushing was required, perineum pain can last longer and require assistance from a pelvic floor therapist for complete recovery.

Cord prolapse, while rare, is said to be increased in a twin delivery. This is where the cord descends before the baby does and can be detrimental to your baby's health. Emergency caesarean is typically required in the event that the prolapse is severe with baby nowhere near ready to descend. In situations where the cord comes out before the baby, but baby is close to delivery, your doctor or midwife can gently tuck the cord back up and help baby navigate down around it.

Vaginal birth can also pose a small risk for your baby in the event that they become stuck or are unable to pass through the vaginal canal. This can happen for a variety of reasons: either your baby's hand, arm, cord, or sac get in the way of their head as they attempt to enter the canal, or they have shifted into a position that is not ideal (think breech or transverse).

Fetal heart monitoring throughout labor (whether constant or intermittent) is encouraged so that your care provider can judge how well your baby is doing as labor progresses. If at any point your baby's heart rate drops, your care provider will determine alternative options depending on the severity and specific situation.

Many women birth babies, and even twins, vaginally with no complications. As with cesareans, complications tend to be the exception and not the rule. If you take anything away from this chapter, let it be that. The birth process is one that should be trusted. Your body should be trusted to do something that it was designed and created to do. I know it is much easier said than done but try not to walk into the birth process with a heart of fear. Having a supportive medical provider that you trust will make this process so much easier. Discuss any fears or concerns with them and talk it all through until you are at a place of comfort with their ability to handle emergency situations and one-off situations.

All women deserve to birth the way they want to with as much respect and support from their attending medical personnel as possible. I share this information, not to instill fear, but to show you that the way your babies enter this world matters. A caesarean section is a major surgery with a lot of risks and one that you should not be pushed into at the convenience of your doctor. It should not be the solution to every twin pregnancy, nor should you at any point feel that it is your only option simply because you are growing two humans. While C-sections have their place as a valuable tool to aid in delivery, it should not be the standard simply because you are carrying two babies.

As I've stated before, it is so important to advocate for yourself and for your babies. Don't take no for an answer, and don't settle for the first doctor that pops up on Google when you type in "OBGYN's near me". Do your research, shop around, and don't stop until you find someone that will respect your wishes and desires.

There are obviously going to be times where the circumstances are extenuating, and some cases in which your body may not be able to safely birth your babies the way you want. These are times for you and your doctor to discuss the pros and cons of each delivery, the risk factors associated with it, and you and your medical professional's comfort level going forward. Whatever path you take in bringing your twins earth side, I hope that you as a woman are supported and respected and presented with all the options that are available.

Chapter 6

Added Care

"Pregnancy is getting company inside one's skin."

Maggie Scarf

As I mentioned in chapter two, there will be moments in the coming months where you will do anything to find a small amount of physical comfort. Where you will happily pay someone all the money if it means that you can breathe deeply without a bum or foot stuck in between your ribs. True story, I once could barely breathe for three days due to twin B being lodged under my rib cage. It was annoying and exhausting, and quite frankly, simply part of this twin pregnancy process. However, there is help, and below I've compiled a list of each resource I sought out during my pregnancy that aided in my comfort and wellbeing. Every moment of comfort and physical relief that can be found while your body and babies grow is worth gold in my humble opinion and I highly encourage you to take advantage of each of these resources and what they have to offer.

Chiropractic Care:

One of my weekly staples was my chiropractor. Dr. Tara Connolly of Sozo Chiropractic was an absolute godsend. I credit her gentle care with keeping me mostly sane and somewhat comfortable for a long as I was.

As with your choice of medical provider, it is important to find a chiropractor that you trust and feel comfortable with who has a proven track record. Ask around, read reviews and do your homework to find someone that is knowledgeable and skilled. Don't let your second cousin who hasn't graduated from chiropractic school give you an adjustment; your body does not need to be a guinea pig at this point in time. You need a skilled chiropractor that is certified in the Webster Technique. They can make a world of difference in your comfort level as your body grows.

The Webster Technique is a specific adjustment to the sacrum that helps align your pelvis and optimizes your nervous system function. It allows the pelvis muscles and ligaments to become more balanced, creating more comfort for you and more space within your womb for your babies to move and grow. This is especially important in a twin pregnancy when your babies require so much more space than a singleton. Pregnancy in general puts a lot of strain on your body, and with a twin pregnancy your body is growing so much faster that sometimes a little bit of help to keep you aligned is needed.

I could always feel such a huge difference in my body before and after an adjustment. My chiropractor specialized in prenatal care, and she always seem to know exactly what tweaks I needed to help with my discomfort.

Dr. Tara was my go-to when Baby B decided to nestle into my lungs for a bit. I could feel her bottom pressing on my left bottom rib. I could barely eat, my chest felt tight, and I was unable to take a deep breath. Dr. Tara had me lay down and made a few adjustments to my round ligaments (the ligaments helping support my uterus). As soon as I stood up after the adjustment, both of my babies shifted down into my pelvis. My round ligaments had become tense from walking and that small adjustment loosened them up so that my hips could expand outward better. It gave my babies more room to settle into my body. For the first time in days I could breathe deeply, and I may or may not have cried when I realized how instant the relief was.

I also credit chiropractic care and the Webster Technique for my babies being in the optimal position for birth. The Journal of Manipulative and Physiological Therapeutics reported in 2002 that there was an 82% success rate of babies turning vertex when the Webster Technique was used in the 8th month of pregnancy, which is past when babies would have typically turned vertex on their own. As we discussed in the previous chapter, your baby's position within your womb can have an impact on your birth options.

I began seeing my chiropractor around 12 weeks pregnant, and continued seeing her at least twice a week, or more depending on my comfort or lack thereof, until I delivered. By 29 weeks, both babies had turned vertex. Her adjustments to my sacrum and round ligaments helped my body function optimally and allowed as much space as possible for my babies to navigate themselves into a position that both of them and my body knew was best.

When used consistently in pregnancy, chiropractic care can be incredibly beneficial for both you and your babies and should not be overlooked as part of your overall care and well-being.

Spinning Babies:

Another helpful tool for you during your pregnancy is a practice called Spinning Babies. Spinning Babies was created by Gail Tully, a midwife who believed that birth could be easier, less painful, and more successful if steps were taken to ensure that your body was in balance and baby was in an optimal position for birth.

The Spinning Babies techniques and logic go hand-in-hand with the chiropractic belief that the body must be aligned and balanced to provide adequate space for your babies as they grow. As your body grows quickly to accommodate two babies, muscles can spasm and joints can become misaligned. Both of these things can cause the uterus to pull out of alignment with the pelvis.

Tully believes that your baby's position within your womb is an indication of the misalignment within your body. She created specific movements and activities that help support and stabilize the pelvis, loosen tight muscles and ligaments supporting the uterus, and balance and align the uterus so that your body finds comfort as it grows, which is her main goal for the mother as pregnancy progresses. With comfort comes a balance within the uterus, and with balance comes your baby's natural instinct to rotate head down. Balancing your body and aligning your uterus and pelvis simply opens your womb up to make more room for your baby to do exactly what they know to do.

This balance and opening up of your body is even more essential in a twin pregnancy than a singleton, in my opinion, and Tully specifically mentions the spinning babies technique in regard to twins on her website. Her advice and practice of balancing the mother to help the babies turn has been a source of guidance for mothers, midwives, and doulas across the world. Even if your provider is comfortable attempting a breech delivery, labor and delivery is easier and safer if your babies are vertex and Spinning Babies is a great place to find techniques to encourage cephalic presentation with both of your babies.

While I will briefly outline some of her techniques here, I highly recommend that you visit Tully's website to get an in depth look at the full instructions regarding the practice of spinning babies. It's easy to remember: https://spinningbabies.com. Navigate to the Menu, and click the Twin link under the Pregnancy tab. Her website also has a wealth of information regarding tutorials for the techniques, as well as personal and anecdotal stories involving full term twin births.

Tully is also an advocate of a healthy diet in pregnancy. She is quoted as saying "Personally, I find twin births to nutritionally well fed and healthy women go quite amazing! If you are well nourished and healthy, and stay healthy through good nutrition for your needs, you are likely to go full term" and she goes as far as to quote Dr. Brewer's advice regarding nutrition in twin pregnancy under the Twins tab of her website. Tully provides information regarding breech and transverse twins, and advice on external cephalic versions (manual manipulation to turn babies). It is a wonderful place to browse for inspiration and positive encouragement in an approach to twin pregnancy.

Spinning Babies Techniques for Twins (Per Gail Tully - Spinning Babies):

Jiggling - also referred to as Manteada, Chunging or Sifting: while on your hands and knees, you place a long piece of fabric comfortably across your belly. Your partner, doula, or midwife stands over you and gently (*gently*) pulls the ends of the fabric up so that your belly is lifted. It briefly lifts the weight of your uterus from your body and allows your hip muscles to loosen. Think of it as a hammock for your belly.

Forward-Leaning Inversion: a move that is highly recommended to be done while being spotted or supported by a partner. Place your knees on a bench or couch, and slowly and carefully lower your hands to the floor. The effect leaves you slightly upside down, and the gravitational pull encourages babies to flip if they have the room to do so.

Maternal Positioning: this is more about maintaining good balance within your body. It follows Tully's technique of Rest Smart, which is the optimal position for rest to maintain good balance. It details to lay with knees lower than your hips, your belly lower than hips, and allowing your lower back to sway forward in stand and walking. Again, the idea is that your belly is to be a hammock for your babies.

Other techniques recommended are the Standing Sacral Release, Abdominal/Diaphragmatic Release, and Side-lying Release. All techniques are designed to be gentle and effective at bringing balance and comfort back to your body to enhance your baby's ability to rotate naturally down into the uterus. Again, please see her website for full instructions on performing these techniques.

As you go through the exercises and activities outlined in Spinning Babies, remember to be gentle with yourself. You are not attempting to force your babies to move. You are simply trying to align your body properly so that they have room to move when they are ready to do so.

Prenatal Massage:

Massage therapy is another wonderful way to find relief as your body stretches and pushes your comfort levels to the max. Massage therapy has not only been proven to be safe while pregnant, but studies have shown that it has many benefits for both mother and baby.

One study in particular conducted by Tiffany Field, director of the Touch Research Institute at the University of Miami Miller School of Medicine, found that regular prenatal massage reduced cortisol (stress) levels, and reduced anxiety. Women who completed the study also reported that their sleep had improved and their overall moods were lightened. Women reported a reduction in back and leg pain, stemming from the weight of their uterus pressing into the nerves and veins.

A few women even reported that massage therapy lessened the effects of prenatal depression. Fields study found that women who completed the massage therapy also had lower incidences of premature labor, though the exact science behind that has yet to be fully explored.

A bonus to massage therapy, in addition to the relaxation of sore muscles, reduced stress and anxiety, and better sleep, is that it can help your blood flow and restore circulation that may be reduced due to strain on your veins. Better blood flow means easier and better nutrient distribution to both you and your baby, which as we've discussed is always a good thing.

Fields not only attributed the relaxing effects of the massage to the positive results, but her aim was to explore the effects that consistent and prolonged human touch had on the comfort and stress levels of a pregnant woman. Her study also noted that women who had regular massages from their partner reported the same positive results as the women who had regular massages from a licensed therapist.

If a professional massage isn't in your budget or schedule, ask your partner for a little extra hands-on affection. It may be something as simple as a foot massage, or a light rub across sore calves, or a simple squeeze across your tight shoulders.

As you get closer to your due date, it is important that you strive to be as relaxed as possible. A woman at ease tends to usher in labor better than a woman who is stressed and anxious about the impending labor process (or subsequent arrivals of TWO newborns). Being in a state of stress can actually delay the onset of labor in some cases. Being able to find comfort and relaxation is so wonderful for your body and state of mind, especially as you near the end of pregnancy. As with chiropractic care, it is important to find someone who is certified in prenatal care. They will know best the positions to put you in that will not add any extra strain or discomfort to your body or babies.

Acupuncture:

Acupuncture is a form of traditional Chinese healing that has been around for thousands of years. It is considered a safe practice in pregnancy, with some claiming that it helps with anything from morning sickness, to back pain, to inducing labor (after safely arriving at your due date).

In acupuncture, hair fine needles are placed at various points in the skin called meridians. These points correspond to nerves in the body and the needles activate the nerves to promote the release of brain chemicals that help with pain.

There have been a few studies that back up the claim that acupuncture can help with nausea, back pain, sleep issues, and depression. A study done in New Zealand should that 89% of woman who underwent acupuncture had a reduction in their pain levels.

Yoga:

If you feel like prenatal yoga has been a bit of a buzzword over the last decade or so, it is because it has been. Yoga is a great low-impact workout that can help ease some of the pains you are experiencing. It can be modified as little or as much as you need to match your personal fitness and comfort levels. It focuses on building balance, strength and flexibility, all of which will be beneficial to you during pregnancy, labor, delivery and life with newborn twins.

Yoga is also a great way to usher in relaxation and let go of stress. It introduces a calming and grounded mindset through gentle, flowing movements and deep breathing exercises. Again, all of which are incredibly beneficial to you from now until the time your twins are eighteen. Being able to tap into a calming breathing pattern is not as easy as it sounds, and it requires practice and patience. By practicing being in a state of calm, you can actually make yourself achieve it as needed.

Yoga is a great tool during pregnancy both mentally and physically. While most times a prenatal yoga routine is considered safe to do while pregnant, it is important to talk to your doctor or midwife for clearance before beginning, especially if you are new to the practice of yoga. Also, it is incredibly important to listen to your body. If anything causes pain or makes you feel uncomfortable, please refrain from the exercise and discuss with your care provider.

Chapter 7

Estimating Risks

"Motherhood is the greatest thing and the hardest thing."

Ricki Lake

This book would not be complete if we did not take a look into the risks associated with a multiples pregnancy. It's easy to assure you that everything will be fine, but the goal is to provide adequate information for you to make an informed decision, and I would be remiss if I did not cover the things that could potentially affect you or your babies' health.

For me personally, I needed to know what we could possibly be facing in our pregnancy. I sought this information out with the belief that having knowledge of the risks would better help me limit those risks. In an odd way, it was comforting and helped reduce my anxiety, especially when I found out how much could be reduced by something as simple as diet.

While it can sound alarming to hear that there is an increase in risks for a twin pregnancy versus a singleton, the level of risk is actually still quite low. Serious complications, such as the ones I've listed below, are fairly rare and typically only affect a small percentage of women pregnant with twins. Please take that to heart and let me say it again: the risks of complications in a twin pregnancy is fairly low. Do not let people make you believe you are a walking bomb simply because it happens more in a twin pregnancy than in a singleton pregnancy. Most of the women I know who have had twins, had healthy pregnancies with no complications.

As stated in our chapter Eating for Three, there are many ways in which your diet can influence some of the risks associated with twin pregnancy that have been backed by science. Along with informing you of the risks you may potentially encounter, I will also offer ways in which you can further lower your chances of complications. Good prenatal care is also a must, as any potential complications that arise can be dealt with early on, or even prevented altogether. Understanding the risks and being aware of their symptoms may seem frightening, but it is essential that you arm yourself with this knowledge. The more you know, the better equipped you will be in making healthy, wise decisions regarding your body, babies, and care.

Preterm Labor:

The most common complication of twin pregnancy is preterm labor. Preterm labor is defined when the mother goes into labor before 37 weeks. Studies show that as many as 60% of twin pregnancies end in preterm labor. If not stopped, the result is premature babies. Babies that come before term struggle much more than babies that are delivered at term, and not just in initial days of life. Some babies can have long term health issues for the rest of their lives. Depending at what stage the preterm labor takes place, the prognosis varies. Thanks to modern day technology, babies born as young as 24 weeks gestation stand a chance at surviving, though it is an uphill climb for both the baby and the parents. Preterm babies will spend a lot of time in a Neonatal Intensive Care unit until certain milestones are achieved.

Some of the risks associated with premature babies are low weight with a tendency to have trouble gaining weight, as their instinct and ability to suckle is hindered. Their lungs can be underdeveloped which results in a slew of breathing issues like apnea and respiratory distress syndrome. Respiratory distress syndrome occurs when babies lack a protein called surfactant and as a result, the small air sacs in their lungs collapse. Premature babies are also more likely to have bronchopulmonary dysplasia, which causes fluid to fill their lungs and can result in scar tissue and damage.

Babies born before term can have trouble regulating their body temperature, which results in needing to be incubated as much as possible. Their hearts can be underdeveloped as well, which can result in many issues, one of which is patent ductus arteriosus. PDA is a result of the ductus failing to close properly after birth leaving a failure of connection between two major blood vessels. In this case surgery is required to repair the ductus. The baby's liver can also suffer as a result of preterm birth which leads to jaundice. Anemia happens when the baby doesn't have enough healthy red bloods cells to carry oxygen to the rest of their body. Brain issues can occur due to the ventricles in the brain being underdeveloped, as well as vision problems due to the retinas and blood vessels being underdeveloped. Preterm babies are also at greater risk of infection due to their immune systems being underdeveloped.

What you can do for prevention:

While preterm labor is indeed the most common complication, I feel that it can be prevented. Again, as stated by Dr. Brewer, Dr. Goodnight and Dr. Newman and supported by numerous experts in the field of multiples, studies have shown that a nutritious diet by the mother can lead to longer gestation. Proper rest, adequate nutrition and hydration have been proven to reduce the likelihood of preterm labor. Every single twin mother that I personally know who has put in the effort to eat a high protein diet has gone on to carry their twins to 39 weeks or longer. Do not let the statistics scare you: many women carry their twins full term and give birth to healthy babies. It is simply a matter of understanding the importance of nutrition in your twin pregnancy and working hard to ensure that you are eating a diet that is conducive to good health.

Intrauterine Growth Restriction (IUGR):

IUGR is typically defined as a slowing or complete stop to one or both of your baby's growth while pregnant. IUGR can happen for a number of reasons, and it tends to happen more in a multiples pregnancy than a singleton. Studies have shown that it occurs in about 10% of twin pregnancies, with monochorionic pregnancies making up the majority of that 10%.

Most providers will require you to have more sonograms and growth scans, particularly the further along you get. If at any point they detect that your babies are not on track or growing as they should be, you might hear this term. IUGR can range from mild to severe, with severe cases being extremely rare. The recommended course of action for mild cases of IUGR are close monitoring.

What you can do for prevention:

Some people believe that IUGR happens because the placentas simply can't keep up with the demand of your growing babies, but I do not believe that to be the case. A healthy diet with a focus on protein and fresh, nutrient rich vegetables, has been proven to help the placenta continue to function at its best. Your body made your babies, and it made your placentas. It is perfectly capable of carrying them too.

Chiropractic care is great way to ensure that your body is functioning optimally. Spinning babies and yoga, or another low impact exercise program, can also be utilized to ensure that your body is in balance and your uterus and pelvis are aligned the way they need to be to better able to accommodate the demands of your babies' growth.

Another thing you can do: try not to worry. Despite all the advances we have when it comes to sonograms and intrauterine imaging, it is still hard to determine a baby's exact size and weight. Unless the growth has stopped completely, it may be hard to tell exactly how off track your baby's growth is by a simple sonogram. Continue eating a healthy diet and try not to stress if one of your babies (or both) look to be on the smaller side.

Twin-to-Twin Transfusion Syndrome (TTTS):

TTTS is a condition that is limited to monochorionic pregnancies (Mo/Mo or Mo/Di) and occurs when one twin begins receiving more nutrients than the other. It is a result of abnormal blood vessels within the placenta that divert and send all the nutrients one way instead of equally between the two umbilical cords. While TTTS can be a serious complication, it is also very rare.

TTTS can occur at any point in your pregnancy, which is why sonograms are recommended more often if your twins are sharing a placenta. If caught early enough, there is a better chance to help combat the severity of TTTS, as there are five different stages.

Stage 1 is mild with the only indicator being that one twin has more amniotic fluid in their sac than the other. At this stage, you will be monitored closely to see if the differences continue to grow. Stage 2 shows an even greater discrepancy between the amount of fluid in each twin's sac, as well as an inability to detect one twin's bladder on the ultrasound. The twin that is not receiving the proper nutrients (referred to as the donor) will see a decrease of intake and output of the amniotic fluid due to the fact that it is not replenishing as it should. The twin receiving more than its share of the nutrients (referred to as the recipient) will have an overabundance of fluid as well as a full bladder. At Stage 3, there is a noticeable difference in the umbilical cords as the blood flow is going to one and not the other. At stage 4, the recipient twin starts showing signs of strain and heart failure due to his body trying to process the overabundance of nutrients, while the donor is showing signs of strain and failure to thrive due to not receiving enough. At this point, the TTTS can be life threatening to both twins. Stage 5 indicates that one twin, either the donor or the recipient, has passed.

In cases of severe TTTS (stages 3-4), your medical provider will probably weigh the pros and cons of early delivery to see if your babies are better off being born early or if they can potentially stand the prolonged strain of TTTS within the womb. At lot of times this while be determined by your current gestation. If you are close to term, the recommendation will probably be early delivery.

While I understand that this can be frightening to hear if your twins share a placenta, the good news is that only 15% of monochorionic pregnancies will develop TTTS. Thanks to modern technology and medical treatment, the vast majority of that 15% survive and the majority of those survivors go on to lead normal lives.

What you can do for prevention:

Dr. Julian De Lia, founder of the Twin to Twin Transfusion Syndrome Foundation, has found that a high protein, nutritious diet has been shown to not only be helpful in possibly preventing TTTS, but can also improve the fetal signs of established TTTS. Not to sound like a broken record, but once again, nutrition is key to helping our bodies and placentas work optimally to ensure our babies grow and develop as best as they can. The nutrients that you provide your body with will go on to help establish a strong and healthy placenta for your babies.

Gestational Diabetes:

Gestational Diabetes is a condition in which you develop diabetes while pregnant. It occurs more often in a twin pregnancy, due to an increase in hormones. While pregnant, your body becomes more resistant to insulin than it normally is, and the extra hormones can cause your body to respond to insulin differently, leading to the condition. It typically goes away after delivery but having this condition can predispose you for other issues such as preeclampsia and preterm labor.

What you can do for prevention:

Gestational Diabetes can be managed, and quite possibly prevented altogether, with a healthy diet and exercise program throughout your pregnancy. Many women go on to have healthy pregnancies and babies while having GD. It is important to discuss nutrition with your doctor or specialist if you are diagnosed with GD to find out specifically how to manage your insulin needs.

Cord Entanglement:

Cord Entanglement will only affect monoamniotic (Mo/Mo) pregnancies. With two babies sharing a sac, kicking and twisting and growing around each other, it is possible that their cords can become intertwined and wrapped around each other. This entanglement can cause your babies to not descend properly into the birth canal due to a lack of room and mobility.

Many obstetricians believe the risk for a vaginal birth is too great and recommend a C-section, as cord entanglement can lead to true umbilical knots when the babies attempt to pass through the birth canal. The severity of entanglement and its impact on your labor and delivery plans should be discussed with your care provider so that you can make an informed decision regarding the best route to proceed.

What you can do for prevention:

Try not to stress! There is not much you can do to prevent your babies from rolling around in your womb. Luckily, the umbilical cord has a thick, cushion-like substance called Wharton's Jelly that helps protect and insulate the blood vessels within the umbilical cord. Even if your little ones have woven themselves together like a tapestry, it is very unlikely that cord entanglement will pose a risk to their overall health. Fetal death due to umbilical knots is extremely rare, thanks to this built-in cushion within the cord. The bigger your babies grow within you, the less room they will have to tango around each other and any intertwining that does occur will likely pose little risk to their development or health.

Placenta Abruption:

Placenta abruption is slightly more common in twin pregnancies; however, the risk is still quite low with studies showing that it only affects about 3% of all twin pregnancies. Placental abruption is when the placenta detaches from the uterine wall before either baby is born. Some doctors believe there is an increased risk of the placenta detaching after twin A is born, but before Twin B can born, especially in a monochorionic pregnancy. Placenta abruption is life threatening to the baby still in utero, and typically requires emergency C-section, or immediate vaginal delivery, to ensure survival of the baby.

What you can do for prevention:

Many midwives believe that clamping the cord of Twin A fairly quickly after delivery reduces the risk of placental detachment. Further studies have shown that the use of alcohol, smoking, and illicit drugs during pregnancy are more significant risk factors for placental abruption than simply carrying twins. Doctors and midwives are trained to watch for signs of placental abruption during labor so if you have a trusting relationship with your care provider you can relax and know that you are in good hands in the event of this rare complication. Again, it must be said, that a healthy diet more often than not lends itself to a healthy placenta. A healthy placenta will continue functioning the way nature intended it to, with placental detachment occurring only after the umbilical cord has stopped delivering blood to your baby, which is typically up to an hour after your baby is born. My twins were born three hours apart, and my placenta stayed attached to the uterine wall throughout my labor and delivery of twin B. My midwife informed me that she once had a mother deliver her twins 13 hours apart without any complications or risk of the placenta detaching.

Cord Prolapse:

Cord prolapse is when the cord of a baby slips down out of the birth canal before the baby does and can cause fetal distress. Once the umbilical cord is exposed to oxygen and room temperature, the Wharton's Jelly begins to shrivel and constrict against the blood vessels within the cord. The temperature outside of your body is significantly lower than that of your uterus. It is part of a natural design to signal to your baby that it's time to take his or her first breath. If the cord is exposed to the cooler temperature before the baby is, and the cord begins to restrict the blood flow, there is a chance that the baby will lose oxygen supply and go into respiratory distress. This can happen in any pregnancy regardless of whether or not you are carrying twins, but it is still quite rare. Some doctors believe that a monoamniotic pregnancy has an increased risk due to the babies sharing a sac. The concern is that twin A, being entangled with the cord of twin B, might bring the cord of twin B out when they are born. This is another reason many doctors and midwives encourage a Caesarean section in the case of Mo/Mo twins.

What you can do for prevention:

Sonograms leading up through the third trimester can indicate whether or not there is cord entanglement. If there is, it is in your best interest to discuss the pros and cons of a vaginal delivery with your care provider. In the case of dichorionic pregnancies, where each baby and their cord are safely tucked into their own sac, the likelihood of cord prolapse is very rare. This is why many midwives and doctors prefer that baby A be head down against the cervix, as this position drastically reduces the risk of the cord slipping down and out ahead of the baby. As previously stated, if the cord happens to slip out before the baby does, but your baby is close to delivery, the cord can simply be tucked back into the body to delay the process of restriction while your baby finishes the birth process.

Preeclampsia:

Preeclampsia is a condition in which you develop high blood pressure and have a high level of protein output in your urine. It is typically marked by sudden weight gain and rapid swelling of your extremities. While it can occur in any pregnancy, it tends to be more common in a twin pregnancy due to the added strain of carrying two babies; however, it is still quite rare with an incidence rate of only 2-5%. If it goes unchecked, it can be dangerous for the mother leading to damage of the organs. However, your care provider should be monitoring your blood pressure and urine at every appointment which helps with early detection. This is another reason that prenatal care with a trusted provider is very important to your pregnancy. Preeclampsia tends to develop in later pregnancy, usually after 37 weeks but it's not impossible to develop before then. The only cure for preeclampsia is delivery of your babies, but if it is a fairly mild case your medical provider may just monitor you closely and recommend rest. Preeclampsia will resolve itself after delivery.

What you can do for prevention:

While much of the medical community still believes the cause of preeclampsia to be unknown, Dr. Brewer's theory from his clinical studies and observations found that women who restricted either protein or calories while pregnant were much more likely to fall victim to this disease. When Dr. Brewer first began looking at nutrition in relation to pregnancy, his end goal was to eliminate preeclampsia, or toxemia as it was called in the 1950's. His studies produced the basis of our information in chapter three regarding nutrition and gestation duration, but this information was just a side note in comparison to his greater goal of finding the cause of preeclampsia in women.

Post-Partum Hemorrhage:

PPH is thought to be slightly greater in a twin pregnancy due to the larger area that the placenta covers along the uterine wall, as well as the overextension of the uterus. After delivery of your babies and placentas, your uterus begins to contract to help restrict blood flow to the vessels where your placenta was connected to the uterine wall. Sometimes, when your uterus has been overextended, it does not contract as well as it should which prevent the blood vessels from constricting properly, thus leaving them to bleed freely which results in hemorrhage. Hemorrhage is classified as losing more than 500ml of blood following birth. Rapid blood loss through hemorrhage can cause a drop in blood pressure which can lead to shock, or even death, if not treated immediately. While it can be a serious complication, early detection and treatment can ensure that it does not become life threatening. It is important that your doctor or midwife is observing your postpartum blood loss closely to ensure that it is normal.

What you can do for prevention:

Some studies have found a correlation between postpartum hemorrhage and your hemoglobin levels. When your hemoglobin levels get too low, you develop anemia. Anemia in pregnancy is a condition in which your blood doesn't have enough healthy red blood cells to carry oxygen and tissues to your babies and your body. It is twice as likely to occur in women who are carrying twins and is usually a result of a lack of iron or other vital nutrients in your diet. Once again, nutrition can come to the rescue to combat anemia. Iron is typically found in dark leafy greens such as spinach and broccoli, as well as legumes (beans, lentils, chick peas, peas), red meat, unrefined whole grains like quinoa, and baked potatoes. Anemia is easily prevented by diet alone, but you can also take iron supplements. Some prenatal vitamins include iron as it is a common deficiency in pregnancy. Your doctor or midwife will typically check your blood in the third trimester to determine your hemoglobin level and take action as needed.

Aside from prevention, postpartum hemorrhage can be managed in the event that it does occur. Pitocin, a synthetic form of oxytocin, is usually administered in this situation to help your body begin contracting. Vigorous uterine massage is also recommended, as it can help the uterus begin contracting to help close the vessels. If blood loss is severe, you may need a transfusion or possibly even surgery to attempt to diagnose the source of bleeding.

In extreme cases, and typically as a last resort, a hysterectomy (surgical removal of the uterus) is recommended. If you are choosing to birth outside of a hospital, postpartum hemorrhage does not necessarily mean an immediate transfer to the hospital. Some midwives keep Pitocin on hand just for hemorrhage situations, and most are practiced in the art of uterine massage as a means to induce contractions. Some midwives even believe that placing a piece of your placenta in your mouth can help slow the bleeding. While the thought may make you queasy, not only do midwives have anecdotal proof that this curbs bleeding immediately, but there have been a few scientific studies that back these claims.

Your placenta is extremely rich in nutrients and hormones such as oxytocin, iron, selenium, fatty acids, and progesterone. It also contains blood-clotting agents called fibrinogen and thrombocytic factions, among many other vitamins. When the oxytocin and fibrinogen are absorbed into your mucus membranes through your mouth, it instantly causes your uterus to contract strongly and the blood vessels to constrict and clot. Chewing or sucking on a piece of your placenta may not appeal to you, but if you are pursuing a non-hospital route of delivery with your twins, it is important that you keep an open mind and rely on the expertise of your midwife in the event that it may be needed. You chose her for a reason, and hopefully your trust in her abilities to handle emergency situations was factored into the choice.

Conclusion:

The purpose of this chapter was not to strike fear in you; rather the opposite. I share this information so that you can realize how important it is to take care of yourself during this essential period of growth. When you understand everything that your body is going through, you better understand the importance of what it needs.

As you can clearly see, a high protein, high calorie diet to keep up with the nutritional demands of a twin pregnancy will go a long way in helping prevent a lot of these risks, as they can be mitigated by diet alone. Rest, exercise, chiropractic care, and relaxation techniques such as massage and yoga can also go a long way to ensure that your body is functioning optimally as you grow and create life.

For the duration of your pregnancy, you have no greater job than to ensure you are doing everything in your power to give your babies the best start to life that you possibly can. This means becoming familiar and knowledgeable regarding the risks, listening to your body, resting as much as necessary, and eating a balanced diet that focuses on giving your body and your babies the nutrition it needs to thrive.

If at any time you feel concerned that you may be developing a complication, please do not hesitate to reach out to your provider. This is where a trusting relationship with your care provider is so helpful. Share your concerns with your doctor or midwife over any potential complication that may arise and make a plan for how you will handle it. Feel empowered to discuss each complication at length and make sure that they address your concerns to your satisfaction.

One of my fears as I got closer to my due date was postpartum hemorrhage, and it really helped to discuss it with my midwife. I was able to get a clear view on her experience with PPH and what we would do should it occur. I became intimately knowledgeable on the causes, prevention and management methods, and our plan of action if it was detected in the aftermath of our birth. Instead of feeling fear, I felt empowered by my knowledge, and it really helped put my mind at ease as we grew closer to our due date. I knew that my midwife could competently handle this situation should it occur, and since she was aware of my fear, she was able to give me constant reassurance after the birth of my twins that my bleeding was not only normal, but fairly minimal.

The whole purpose of this book is to help you find confidence and peace as you walk this road. As a woman and a mother, I want you to feel strong and empowered to face this pregnancy with knowledge and a sense of peace.

Chapter 8

Embracing the Emotions

"To be pregnant is to be vitally alive, thoroughly woman, and distressingly inhabited. Soul and spirit are stretched – along with body – making pregnancy a time of transition, growth, and profound beginnings."

Anne Christian Buchanan

When I was 26 weeks pregnant with our twins, I woke one morning feeling a bit of discomfort. I couldn't quite put my finger on it, but a low pain was radiating through my lower abdomen. After a few seconds, it went away. Three minutes later, it came back. I panicked. I immediately thought I was having contractions. I called my midwife who advised me to go to the ER. My husband was stuck in a meeting with vendors who had flown in specifically for this occasion and was unable to come meet me, so I gathered my then 18-month-old and rushed to the hospital by myself.

The nurses quickly got me set up in the labor and delivery unit and strapped on heart monitors to see how our babies were doing, while another monitor was tightened around my belly to view my contractions. Visions of premature babies swam in my head as I hoped and prayed that I wasn't in labor.

My 18-month-old was wandering around the hospital room by himself, and before I could stop him, he ran into the adjoining bathroom and shut the door, where I quickly realized he was unable to get himself out. I was strapped into the bed in seven different ways and unable to move the three feet necessary to open the door for him. As I pressed the call button to ask the nurse to come and free my toddler, I felt the tears pricking at my eyes as doubt flooded my mind.

How in the world was I going to do this? How could I possibly keep up with this rambunctious toddler and two new babies? Where would I find the time, the energy, the space in my heart? How in the world was this going to work? I had a moment where I allowed pity to creep in, where I let the fear settle over me. The nurse graciously came to open the door for my son, and he ran to me and crawled onto my lap. I stroked his hair and felt like I was somehow already failing. Failing to protect him. Failing to keep our babies safe in my body. Failing at motherhood in general as I pondered how thin I could stretch before breaking wide open, physically and metaphorically.

As I wallowed in pity, a cramp darted across my stomach once more, and it was at that moment that I realized my contractions were not contractions at all. I was suffering not from premature labor, but a case of painful gas. While the relief was immense (no pun intended), I also felt slightly mortified for not knowing the difference between labor contractions and gas. Shortly after that, I was released to go home where I promptly snuggled up with my son and took a long afternoon nap. The timeliness of my gas cramps seemed like a sign from the universe. A sign to breathe and accept. To let go of my perceived failings and embrace the moment. It felt like a sign telling me that everything was going to be okay. A silly sign, if you ask me, but who am I to question the universe?

The emotional toll is something that I feel must be addressed. Finding out you are expecting twins can be a surprise, to say the least. There are many factors to consider when you are bringing life into this world, and when it's twins the worries, fears, and burdens can be amplified exponentially. You realize that two babies mean two everything. Two cribs. Two car seats. Another car if two car seats don't fit in your current one. Twice the diapers. Twice the clothes. And on the list goes.

Some women feel nothing but joy and excitement from the moment they realize they are expecting twins. To those women, I salute you and I am happy that you were immediately welcoming of this incredible gift. Other women, like me, may need a little time and encouragement to get there.

I remember the moment I found out that we were expecting not one, but two, little babies. I can close my eyes and suddenly I'm back in the darkened room with my husband at my feet and my toddler curled beside me on the table. The moment the ultrasound wand touched my stomach, I saw it. Two perfect sacs, side by side. Two babies growing in the space where I expected one. The feelings I felt in that moment were so strong that I will never forget them. Denial. Shock. Fear. Joy. All zipping through my veins at lightning speed, leaving me breathless and speechless.

I immediately sat up and desperately said "No. This can't be right." Hello, Denial. At the technicians urging, I laid back down and began crying as all the *what if's* and *what now's* overwhelmed my mind. Hello, Fear. I stared at the screen as we zoomed in on each baby, getting closer looks at their measurements and development. I felt my body shake uncontrollably as I lay helpless on the table. Hello, Shock. Then a beautiful sound filled the room with a soft *whomp whomp whomp whomp* at 145 beats per minute. Their hearts, beating in sync with each other, nestled right beneath my own. Hello, Joy.

I spent the rest of the day laughing and crying, sometimes at the same time. It felt like I was dancing on a fine line of barely concealed hysteria, and honestly, that feeling didn't go away for some time. It took me months to fully embrace what I had been given. There were healthy doses of happiness, fear, disbelief, anxiety, excitement, and incredulity as I worked to process our new reality.

The healthiest thing I did for myself in those early months was give myself permission to feel whatever I needed to feel without shame or guilt. It's easy to get swept up in the thought that you should be immensely grateful for the gift of twins. After all, many women across the world sacrifice so much for the chance just to have one baby, much less two, and a part of me felt incredibly guilty that I wasn't overjoyed where another woman might have been. However, I had to let the guilt go. My twins came to me because they were supposed to, and in time, I embraced it. The guilt served no purpose in my life or emotional well-being but being allowed to feel fear at the thought of welcoming two lives to mine helped me overcome it in due time.

It's so important to recognize your feelings, whatever they may be, and let yourself feel them. If being pregnant with twins is filling you full of fear, feel it. Feel the frustration. Feel the tension. Feel the stress and anxiety. Embrace the messy and hard feelings. You are not less of a mother, or less of a woman, if the first feelings that surround you at this news isn't joy. You are not less of a person if gratitude is not the first thing that comes to mind. Having a baby is life changing. Having two babies is the equivalent of setting sail to sea in a boat with no oars. Life is about to get beautiful *and* chaotic. There is joy and there is fear. You will have to give more of yourself than you have ever given before. You are allowed to feel *less than*. Less than thrilled. Less than excited. Less than overjoyed.

When I let myself feel the complicated emotions, I let myself process it in a healthy and mindful way. I invited the fear in and gave it a face. I courted the anxiety and gave it name. I sat quietly with the stress and bit by bit, it became less and less overwhelming. I allowed myself to mourn the pregnancy I had envisioned, and the second child I had expected. My life was completely changing in a way I did not anticipate and was not fully prepared for. In order to become prepared, I needed to let myself grieve, heal, and grow. As the months went on, my fear, anxiety, and stress started to give way to excitement, joy, and acceptance. I dealt with my emotions head on and doing so allowed me to embrace the path that lay before me.

Finding a supportive ear can be helpful for sorting through these emotions too. Your partner should be someone that you feel safe to confide in, and a close friend, your mother, or your midwife may be better able to relate specifically to you as a woman. A trusted confidante can provide a good outlet for releasing your fears and anxieties. Talking through some of the things that overwhelm you can make them seem a little less overwhelming. The key here is to find someone who will be supportive and allow you to express your feelings without judgement. You need a safe place that will offer advice and support. Most areas have a Moms of Multiples group that you can join where you can connect with other women who have all walked in your shoes. Social media offers a wealth of support with wonderful groups like Birthing Multiples Naturally on Facebook where fears, worries, and concerns can be expressed with other twin moms.

Wherever you are at now emotionally is exactly where you need to be. Grieve your expectations if that's what you need to do. Get to know your fear intimately and let yourself grow from the interaction. Peace and acceptance are your end goals, and as you work through all your emotions, you will find yourself making peace with them and your situation. Believe me when I say it will all be okay. I cried endless tears throughout my pregnancy. Partly from the hormones, partly from fear, and partly from simply feeling overwhelmed. It was hard to see the big picture, at times, and hard to feel like anything, much less everything, would work out. But it did. Everything worked out for me, and everything will work out for you too. Before you know it, you will find yourself full of so much love for your babies. You won't be able to imagine life without them and these days of fear and overwhelming worry and anticipation will feel like a distant dream.

Prenatal Depression:

It is natural and understandable to feel stress, fear, and anxiety over the impending arrival of twins. However, if you believe that the things you are feeling are not normal or extend beyond the typical concerns and anxieties of pregnancy, I highly recommend that you speak to your care provider as soon as possible. Prenatal depression is very real and can become dangerous for both mother and baby. Signs and symptoms of prenatal depression include:

-persistent sadness. A feeling of sadness that does not let up at all.

-difficulty concentrating on everyday tasks.

-loss of interest in activities that you once enjoyed.

-recurring thoughts of death or suicide.

-extreme anxiety, panic attacks, etc.

If you experience any of the above, please do not be afraid to seek help.

Chapter 9

Calming your mind: Power in Positivity

"Attitude is a little thing that makes a big difference."
Winston Churchill

In chapter 8, we talked about accepting and dealing with the messy emotions that can come from finding out you are having twins. In this chapter, I would like to share ways in which you can center yourself to find peace, positivity, and calm along this journey.

I strongly believe in the power of positivity. I believe that when you purposefully seek out silver linings and half-full glasses, your mindset shifts to see the good in every situation. Walking through your pregnancy with peace and positivity may not come naturally to you, especially when you are tired and aching all over and your mind is a mess from coming to terms with the two new humans you are growing. However, deliberately striving to find positive moments and aspects of this phase of life can be greatly beneficial to you, both now and in the long run.

When you seek and embrace positivity, your own energy - that vital life force inside you - begins vibrating at a higher frequency and in turn it begins to have an effect on every aspect of your life, both inside and out. If there is ever a time to embrace the power of positivity and the ways it can benefit both your mind and body, now would be that time.

Meditation, yoga, and journaling can be very helpful tools in navigating your way through the chaos of your mind and starting you on the path to positivity and gratefulness. Carving out a little time every day to reflect on your babies and your birth can help you bond with them. Find a method that works for you and make it a priority to engage yourself in deliberate and intentional reflection. Envision meeting your little ones for the first time. Envision the first cries and the moment that your eyes will meet theirs. That is the destination of this first leg of a very long journey. That is the moment to keep in mind when everything aches, and your heart is heavy, and you are so over your pregnancy. Visualize your birth down to the specifics, no detail is too small to imagine.

Deep breathing is a great tool to utilize when you start to feel anxiety and stress. I learned to place a hand over my heart, and a hand over my growing belly and take deep, mindful breaths to ground me and connect myself to my little ones. It was during these intentional moments throughout the day that peace started coming to me. It was slow at first, but the better I became at recognizing my feelings of being overwhelmed, the better I was able to combat it with mindful relaxation. It was during these deep breathing exercises that I first began harnessing the power of positivity and using it combat the negativity in my mind.

I also kept a pregnancy journal while carrying my twins. It's amazing now to go back and read the things that were on my mind and heart while in that stage of life. Most of the things I worried about have resolved themselves. The aches and the pains disappeared, and in their place are two beautiful little babies. Writing has always been an outlet for me to process my emotions, so it's natural that it is what I would turn to. However, not everyone wants to write or journal. The key is to find a healthy outlet that lets you process your emotions while also distracting you a bit. If you're a painter, paint. If you like music, immerse yourself in something that brings you to a calm place. If you like crafting, or building, or pottery, let the power of your creativity and the craft of your hobby be your outlet for organizing your thoughts.

In many ways, your twin pregnancy and the following years with newborn, infant, and toddler twins is going to be about simply surviving. Making it through to the next day, the next milestone, sometimes even to the next hour. While this is a beautiful journey, it is also a hard journey and the best way to approach it is with a sense of positivity and optimism.

In talking with a friend of mine, who recently discovered she was expecting twins, we got onto the subject of positivity, specifically in reference to twins and twin pregnancy. She explained that she meditated every night her positive intentions in delivering full term twins that were healthy. I was thrilled to hear this and shared with her that when I was in her shoes, I too meditated daily on the outcome of my twin pregnancy. I envisioned my twins being delivered vaginally, with no medical intervention, after a full-term pregnancy. I wanted this outcome so desperately that I spoke it out loud, I visualized it day in and day out, I wrote it down in my journal, and I meditated on it whenever fear and doubt would try to steal my peace of mind. It became my mantra, and this positive outcome that I kept pushing out into the universe and speaking into being was a lifeline to me whenever I felt overwhelmed by the "what-ifs" that can come with the unknown.

I believe that this positivity radiated out of me and served to free my mind from negativity and worry. The physical burden of twin pregnancy may not have lightened, but having a positive attitude made me see the aches and pains in a different light. I began to accept them as part of a vital journey to having healthy babies and it made me feel grateful instead of resentful. My huge belly that drew looks and not always considerate comments was a sign that my babies were growing big. My back ache was a sign that my body was giving this pregnancy my all. I believe that my positivity in these circumstances made a world of difference in my outlook and outcome, and every positive mantra and desire for my pregnancy and birth came to fruition.

My positive intentions that I focused on for the duration of my pregnancy were as follows: I wanted to go as close to 40 weeks as possible. Ideally, 39 weeks but I would be happy with anything past 37 weeks. I wanted to wake up fresh from a good night's sleep and have labor start first thing in the morning. I wanted to go into labor on a weekend so my husband wouldn't be in the middle of getting ready for work/commuting, and for the ease of our parents being able to come witness the births. I wanted the labor to be relatively short – 6 hours start to finish. I wanted healthy babies with no need for medical interventions or transfers.

Every single day of my pregnancy, I mindfully and willfully put these desires out into the universe. I whispered them to myself while cradling my growing stomach. I wanted as much as possible to speak it into existence.

The reality of our pregnancy and births were almost completely identical to my positive intentions: I went into labor two days shy of 39 weeks. I was in the window of gestation that I had wanted to be in. I woke up at 8:30 after a good night's rest and went into labor around 45 minutes later. It was a Sunday morning - my husband was home and our parents were readily available to pack up and come. The time between the first contraction to our twin B being in my arms was less than five and a half hours. Both babies and I were healthy and required no medical interventions. We were headed home just a few hours after birth.

There is power in positivity. I believe that if you set your mind on all the things that can go right, you will find things going right. If you envision a healthy and positive outcome to your pregnancy, you are setting the expectation into the universe.

If harnessing positivity and the law of attraction is a new concept for you, I urge you to read a few of the following books to help you get started.

The Law of Attraction Plain and Simple by Sonia Ricotti

The Secret by Rhonda Byrne

Positive Thinking: Overcome Negativity and Become a Happier, More Positive Person by Jane Aniston

Chapter 10

Ease and Flow

"Motherhood is the biggest gamble in the world...It's huge and scary – it's an act of

infinite optimism."

Gilda Radner

As we all know, sometimes in life, our best laid plans do not come to be. I think this chapter is necessary and important in keeping with the holistic and mindful approach to pregnancy, even though it feels like the hardest to write.

You can do everything "right". You can eat the healthiest, most nourishing foods, and keep your body well hydrated. You can choose the best prenatal care for yourself and your babies and get adjusted every week only to have something unexpected happen that throws all your plans askew.

When faced with challenges that cause you to suddenly shift gears, particularly if it happens in late pregnancy, it is so important to remember to go with the flow. If Twin A does a flip at 36 weeks and suddenly disqualifies you for your birth with your chosen provider, or a high blood pressure reading suddenly starts looking like preeclampsia, it is important to remember that healthy babies is your ultimate goal. That is not to say that the journey to that destination does not matter, because it does, but sometimes we have to let go of the ideal and embrace the chaos.

It is important to ground yourself in the knowledge that you are doing and have done everything in your power to give your body and babies what they need to flourish. I hope with the information I have provided in this book you will be able to adjust your plans, know your options, and advocate for yourself even in the face of adversity or unforeseen circumstances.

A sweet fellow twin mom that I know was championing to have her twins born out of the hospital. All was going well until 38 weeks. A spike in her blood pressure and her twin B turning breech suddenly disqualified her for her birth center birth with her midwife. She scrambled to find another doctor that would be comfortable attempting to vaginally deliver her twins, and she found one not too far from her home. She had to adapt her plans at the last minute, and though she was not able to birth her twins outside of a hospital setting, she was able to have them vaginally, with few interventions. She now has healthy and happy twin boys.

If you have chosen your medical provider with care and you trust their judgment, then you should continue trusting that their wishes align with yours and they have your best interest at heart, even if the plans you have made together start to unravel.

All this to say, make a Plan A. Do everything you can to achieve it and set it in your mind and heart as the primary option but allow for the possibility of needing a Plan B. Pregnancy, labor, and delivery can all be unpredictable at times, especially in a twin pregnancy when there are many different variables to consider. Sometimes things will happen that are outside your control, but it will be your ability to gracefully adapt that will determine the tone with which it all ends. Stay positive, stay true to yourself and your visions, and remember that all of life eases and flows.

Chapter 11

The Birth of H & T

"Giving birth and being born brings us into the essence of creation, where the human spirit is courageous and bold and the body, a miracle of wisdom."

Harriette Hartigan

This chapter is extremely personal and dear to my heart. In it, I want to share the story of the birth of my twins. It was as close to the birth I had envisioned as I could have hoped for.

On a sunny Sunday morning in July, I woke up feeling refreshed. I had slept until 8 and felt like I had as much rest as possible, considering that I was feeling roughly like the size of a small whale. I was almost 39 weeks pregnant and it was a hundred degrees outside, so I was not much in the mood to get out of the house or do anything other than rest. As I got up and moved to the living room where I was expecting to spend most of the day, I felt a bit of leakage. I shrugged it off, changed my pants, and a few minutes later experienced it again. It started to dawn on me that my water had broken.

By now it was 9 am. I sent my midwife Kim Daly of the Grapevine Birthing Center a message describing the leak and she gave me a few suggestions to encourage contractions to start since I hadn't had any yet. At 9:12 she texted "well let's have some babies today!" Having my suspicions confirmed I told my husband to get ready - they were coming! At 9:15 I then called my mom who was two hours away, and my husband called his parents. While on the phone I had one mild contraction. My mom and my dad were going to head our way, "but don't rush," I told them. I had been in labor for 17 hours with my first child, so I wasn't sure what to anticipate this time around. I contacted my doula, Kelly Martin of The Witty Womb, and our photographer Alyson Osborn of Aly Renee Birth Photography.

At this point, 9:30, my contractions started in earnest. I pulled out my contraction app, sat on my birth ball, and began breathing. By 9:45, just 15 minutes after contractions started, I knew things were going faster than with my first. My contractions were a minute and a half apart and lasting 45 seconds each.

For those unfamiliar with labor and birth, contractions coming a minute apart and lasting for a minute are usual indications that delivery is near. I just didn't think that could be right, as my mind wasn't keeping up with my body. I decided to jump in the shower for mental clarity. I needed to breathe, relax, and reset. The hot shower felt amazing and I stayed in there for close to thirty minutes, breathing and contracting and preparing myself for the day ahead while meditating once more on my ideal labor.

When I got out, I reset my contraction timer and started getting dressed but I could barely focus through contractions at this point. Ten minutes later, barely an hour after my first contraction, I knew things were going fast. Too fast. Contractions were still consistently a minute and a half apart and lasting for 45 seconds to a minute.

I should have known at that point just how close we were, but it didn't dawn on me until a moment later when my contractions started back to back, double peaking with no breaks in between. I was feeling pressure down really low. I realized right then what was happening; I was in transition, which is the point in labor where the cervix is completely dilated, and your baby begins to descend into the birth canal. Meaning, we were moving quickly towards delivery. I was shocked, but also sure. I knew my body and I was certain that we were very close to having a baby.

"We have to leave now. Get Oliver dressed. We have to get to the birth center." I told my husband. As he loaded the truck with Oliver and our birth bag, I took a few minutes to breathe. The contractions had stopped. I felt an uncanny sense of peace fall over me. I knew, I felt it in my heart and in my body, I was fully dilated and that at any minute the urge to push would come over me.

At 10:45, as I was climbing into our truck, it came. I held onto the door frame, threw my head back and let loose a very primal grunt with my contraction as the urge to "bear down" took hold. We were so close to having a baby in our arms. I knew that if we didn't leave right at that moment, we may not make it. I told my husband to drive. We had to get to the birth center right away.

Kim called us as we careened out of our neighborhood, after receiving a text from me that simply said "I have to push". I was in the passenger seat on my knees, facing the back seat. As I answered, a guttural moan came out and the urge to push returned. Kim told me to breathe deeply and get to the birth center ASAP. She told William to put on the flashers and drive as fast as possible.

As another contraction hit me, I told Kim the obvious: "they are coming!" She asked if we needed to pull over and said she could come to us. She could hear it in my voice that I was close to delivery. I took a deep breath and looked at the parking lot of the Wal-Mart we were flying by. *My babies are not going to be born in a parking lot,* I thought with disdain. Little did I know that a parking lot was exactly where one of my babies were about to be born. "We'll be there in ten minutes. William drive faster!" I said through clenched teeth, while fiercely resisting the urge to push.

Kim told us she'd meet us downstairs at the birth center and I went ahead and disconnected. Between my startled and freaked out toddler, my speeding and panicked husband, and the overall urge to push Henry onto the seat of the truck I needed to have one less distraction.

Somehow, someway, we pulled into the parking lot of the birth center about 11:10 am. I saw Kim running to meet us and I took a deep breath and let my body completely relax. We almost made it.

As Kim opened my door another contraction hit me, and I moaned low and deep and I felt Henry fully descend. I was stepping down out of the truck when I felt the ring of fire: the fiery feeling of my baby's head stretching my body wide as his head crowned. William had run around the truck to help me out and I knew he and Kim were right there to catch Henry. I grabbed the handle of the truck and shouted, "he's crowning!"

It seemed like sudden chaos around me. Kim was telling William to get my panties off and telling me to get back in the truck (which was impossible at this point). I don't even remember pushing, I don't remember making any noise, I just remember standing on the running board of the truck, holding the handle and suddenly there he was. My beautiful Baby A, my sweet Henry, crying and stretching his arms out in a move that suggested he was as shocked as we were.

William caught him and was trying to untangle him from my panties. I felt calm, happy, and in complete disbelief as I reached down to grab him. "I got him!" I said as I brought him up to my belly, which was as far as his cord could reach. Someone asked if I was sure I had him, and I was. I knew he was perfectly safe in my hands, even as I hovered a foot off the concrete under an already hot July sun.

As William supported me on the running board, Kim came around to the driver's seat to clamp and cut Henry's cord. He was wailing that beautiful newborn cry as I brought him all the way up to my chest. His cries were mirroring Oliver's, who at this point was still strapped into his car seat in the backseat. "Someone get Oliver!" I shouted, because somehow in that moment he was the one I was worried about. Because I'm a mom.

Someone asked if anyone had caught the time and the reply came back: 11:11. Less than two hours after labor started, and in a parking lot; my son sure knew how to make an entrance. William helped me onto solid ground and made sure I was stable before turning to get Oliver.

It was in that moment that I realized just how panicked my husband was. His hands were shaking, and he was dripping in sweat. I looked around and realized there was blood everywhere, including all over him. It seemed strange to see him upset as I was feeling calm and collected. Unlike my husband, I was riding high on an oxytocin rush, which is a common feeling following a natural birth as your body is flooded with the "love hormone" without anything to dampen it.

"Let's get upstairs before Thea comes!" Was the general consensus and as I started making my way to the back door of the birth center, I caught sight of myself in the reflection of a window. My dress was still bunched around my waist. My pink panties that were now red with blood had hastily been slipped back on. There was blood and afterbirth running down my legs, I was carrying a pink vernix covered fresh-as-could-be crying baby and grinning ear-to-ear. I'll never forget how crazy beautiful fierce I felt in that moment.

I stood in the birthing suite holding Henry and saw that it had been ten minutes since he came. I was eagerly hoping that Thea would join us soon. My mom and dad had arrived by this point, and my dad took Oliver so we could continue to labor. I handed Henry to William and stripped down so I could get into the birth tub. Though contractions had not started back up, the water still felt soothing against my body. I rubbed my legs clean and settled in, unsure of what to expect.

Sensing that we had a bit of time before Thea came, William stepped into the bathroom to shower and change while my mom brought Henry over to me in the tub. I took him and held his little body against me and marveled at the fact that he was here in my arms. I attempted to nurse him and was happy that he latched quickly and eagerly. His suckling spurred a few contractions to start rolling in and I handed him back to my mom so I could meditate and will Thea to join us.

The room was quiet, calm, and filled with a sense of patient waiting as I rolled in the tub and met each contraction with hopefulness. Kelly jumped in and got a cold rag for my face and neck and did hip squeezes that brought such a feeling of relief to my aching back. Each wave brought back pain more than anything and the counter pressure on my hips was heavenly. William joined me by the tub and whispered words of love and encouragement as I calmly breathed through each contraction. My mom snuggled our precious baby A and occasionally brought him over to me during lulls between contractions.

After a few more contractions Kim suggested we get out of the tub and attempt walking to spur Thea into descending. She was still head down and her heart tones sounded strong. It had been over an hour since Henry was born and the time was surprisingly moving fast. I got out of the tub and slipped into a sexy adult diaper, because birthing babies is glamorous like that. A contraction hit me as I was standing, and it was a bit more intense than what I had been experiencing. I turned to the closest person to me, Kelly, and leaned my head on her shoulder. She was soothingly whispering in my ear and coaching me to breathe through the wave since I was suddenly feeling a wave of panic at the pain. I felt intensely grateful for her presence in that moment and I knew my mood was starting to reflect the next level of labor we were entering.

My mom brought me Henry, and William sat and wrapped his arms around me as I nursed our new little baby and breathed through contractions. It continued on like this for another hour. Tara, the in-house chiropractor came upstairs to adjust me, hoping that would help with progressing labor. My bag of waters for Baby B was bulging and it was creating a lot of pressure in my back and the adjustment felt great as it loosened my sacrum and hips.

As badly as I wanted to just push her out, I knew my body wasn't there yet. We went ahead and moved into the bathroom where I sat backwards on the toilet. Someone got me a pillow to lean against and Kim pushed little stools under my feet to put me in a good squat/labor position. Kelly suggested we turn off the lights and the room became quiet as it was just me, Kelly, and Kim. Each contraction in this position got me closer and closer and I started feeling the need to push. My eyes were closed, and I focused on breathing and visualizing Thea moving down, down, down.

As helpful as this position was, my gentle pushes weren't doing much. I didn't know what was going on exactly, but I knew she wasn't coming down like she should have been. At some point, Kim suggested we move to the bed.

"Can I get back in the tub?" I asked, longing for the comfort of the water. Kim gently told me that probably wasn't our best bet since Thea was being stubborn. She really wanted me to get on my hands and knees on the bed, and I trusted her completely. I had a peanut ball under my arms and chest, and I rocked my body through each contraction. I pushed my heart out, leaning back and giving it my all. I used my mom and mother-in-law's hands as leverage - tugging on them while leaning back and pushing, and

William and Kelly started working together to provide amazing relief through my back and hips.

I pushed for what seemed like twenty or thirty minutes, but nothing was happening. She wasn't coming. I heard some talk behind me, then Kim told me she was going to break my water and that when she did, I needed to push and get Thea out. I didn't know what was happening at the time, but I later learned that Thea's heart rate had dropped. My next contraction came, I felt a pop then an immediate feeling of relief as amniotic fluid burst out of my body. The intense pressure was gone, and I pushed, one hand holding my mom and one hand holding my mother-in-law. And suddenly she was out. Three hours and ten minutes after her twin brother had been born, Thea was here. Kim told me that she was handing Thea up to me from between my legs and I reached down to grab her as I sat back.

I'll never forget what happened next. I knew immediately that something was wrong. I brought her to my stomach and said "Hi Thea" as I started rubbing her. But she did not respond. She did not cry. She was completely limp, her skin was white, her lips were blue.

"Thea?" I said, feeling my voice waver as I rubbed her more briskly. "Kim?" There was a definite wobble to my voice as I called out to my midwife. Suddenly Kim was beside me, up on the bed, taking Thea and immediately breathing into her mouth. The other midwives were in action, pulling out an oxygen tank with a mask.

The room burst into motion as time slid to a halt. It was as if everything were in slow motion. I felt William behind me whispering calming words, Kelly was whispering in my right ear that she was okay, some babies just needed help transitioning to life outside the womb.

Panic raged in my heart as I stared at my sweet, unresponsive baby, who was so sickeningly limp. I looked around the room - my mother and mother-in-law were clutching each other. Kim was using a device to suck fluid out of her throat and lungs, as the other midwives prepped the oxygen mask. I took solace in the fact that Thea was still connected to me. Her cord was pumping oxygenated blood into her body and Donna, a seasoned and wise attending midwife, kept reassuring us all that her heart rate was strong. Donna looked at me and said "she's okay. She'll be fine."

She was making raspy noises, not quite breaths, but it was something. It was a start. I trusted my midwife. I trusted her with my life, and with the life of all three of my babies. Despite my fear, I told myself to take comfort in her words.

I reached for Thea, wanting desperately to hold her but I was afraid of interfering. I rubbed her arm and talked to her. "Thea, breathe for mommy. Mommy's right here." Kim told me to keep talking to her, that she was responding to my voice and touch. I kept touching her tiny arm, kept begging her to breathe and cry.

Then, suddenly, I heard her take a breath. And then another. Her face began to take on color. Then she was screaming. And in that moment, it was the most beautiful sound in the world. I sank against William, ugly crying with relief. The whole room seemed to breathe a huge sigh. Kim immediately reached over and unsnapped my bra. "We need to get her skin to skin."

My screaming baby girl was placed against my breasts and a warmed towel and heating pad was laid over us both. She was beautiful. Red faced and squalling, mad as hell, but breathing and beautiful.

I later learned that Thea simply experienced something called birth asphyxia, which studies show can affect 1 in 10 babies at birth. It is when they are born unresponsive. In our particular case, thanks to the experience of our midwives, we had a happy ending. Thea's asphyxia did not cause any short- or long-term issues, due mainly in part to the fact that our midwives kept her connected to the placenta for the sole purpose of receiving the rich oxygenated blood flow to her brain and heart.

In a hospital setting, the typical procedure in dealing with birth asphyxia is to remove the baby from the cord and its mother to be taken to a resuscitation station that is designed for this specific instance. While both methods work, I am grateful that she was kept close to me and connected to her placenta. The midwives did everything that a hospital would have done, they simply did it in proximity to me which studies have shown are more beneficial for a baby that is showing signs of distress. When a baby is already in distress, removal from the smells and sounds of its mother can be even more distressing. I believe that her closeness to my voice and touch had a positive impact on her as she struggled to get that first breath.

While it was a terrifying situation, and one that I hadn't even thought to prepare for, I was once again reminded that my midwives were professionals who were trained for this type of emergency, and my trust in their capabilities helped ease my fear as they worked hard to bring Thea through it.

Soon after Thea was placed on my chest, I birthed the placentas. They had fused together and were in the shape of a heart. At two days shy of 39 weeks, my placentas were in excellent condition and showed no signs of tears or disintegration. The fusion of the two was seamless, and each placenta was rippled with thick, healthy veins. It was another wonderful sign that my body was strong and capable. That our bodies as women are strong and capable.

Start to finish, my labor was five hours long, my babies were healthy, and our labor and delivery had been intervention free (aside from Thea's resuscitation). Everything I had meditated for our birth came to fruition.

Henry was brought back in to us and William did skin to skin with him, and I asked that Oliver be brought in to meet his new siblings. As the five of us curled up on the bed together I couldn't help but feel joy - a wild, heart stopping feeling of love and happiness at my beautiful family. We were in the same room that Oliver had been born in two years before, with two of the same midwives. I was proud of my body for carrying our babies for almost 39 weeks, and for laboring hard to bring them into the world. I had three great births, and three beautiful healthy children. I was grateful for my birth team who reacted calmly and professionally to not one, but two crazy births and who worked hard to ensure that both births had a good outcome. I felt strong, supported, loved, and respected. This is exactly how birth should be.

Chapter 12

The 4th Trimester: Life with Newborn Twins

"There are moments which mark your life. Moments when you realize nothing will ever be the same and time is divided into two parts -before this, and after this."

John Hobbes

Congratulations! You have made it to the other side. This is truly a magical time. These newborn days are fleeting and bittersweet, and I swear there's a little bit of pixie dust in there somewhere. You are getting know the two humans that you grew inside your body and it is such a beautiful journey. As you drift along in the fog that can be post-partum, you may be wondering *what now?*

Now, you just enjoy this ride for what it offers and learn to navigate this path that is parenthood.

There is no wrong way to parent. I mean, there are some obvious wrong ways to parent. I once saw a YouTube video of a two-year-old chain-smoking cigarettes, and I hope we can all agree what category *that* falls into. But when it comes to the little things like formula vs breastmilk or co-sleeping vs sleep training, I think it is important to remember that these are your children and you know what's best. We were given instincts, as mothers and fathers, and I feel that our instincts are usually pretty spot on. I think it's important to follow your instincts while seeking support from your partner. I don't plan to go into too much depth in this chapter regarding the little things, but I will try to offer some insight on how to handle sleeping, feedings and outings with twins.

Bottle vs. Breast:

It matters little where you stand on the proverbial battleground that can be the formula versus breastfeeding debate. I do not judge either way. What matters is that you receive the support you need for the decisions you make. I'm a breastfeeding, co-sleeping, Mom and have been since my first child. However, I know not every mother makes the same decisions I do and that is perfectly okay. There is beauty in our diversity, and every woman deserves to be respected for making what she feels is the best decision for herself and her children.

Regardless of whether you breastfeed or formula feed, a good indication that your baby is getting enough to eat is how often they are filling their diapers. As long as you are changing a wet diaper every few hours, then more than likely they are receiving what they need. Weight gain is also a good indication. While some babies gain slow and some babies gain fast, they should always be gaining weight. Between birth and a few days postpartum, it is not unusual for your baby to lose a few ounces; however, by two weeks old they should be back at their birth weight.

My advice to formula feeding moms of multiples is have their bottles clean and ready for feeding, especially in the early days. One twin mother I know preps an entire day's worth of bottles and keeps them in the fridge so that they can quickly be pulled out and warmed up when it's time to eat. Having your twin's food prepped and quickly produced can help reduce stress around meal times, as a hungry baby is rarely a patient baby.

A bonus of bottle feeding is that your partner can be a part of the feeding experience, which can be valuable bonding time that many partners enjoy having. If you anticipate handling feedings solo, I recommend staggering their eating schedule so that you can feed and burp one before feeding and burping the other.

If you prefer to have your twins eat at the same time both for time efficiency and to keep them on the same schedule, you can invest in bouncy chairs for your babies to sit in while you feed them their bottles. It is important to make sure that the chair adds support to their heads and necks and keeps them at a forty-five-degree angle. Ideally, you want their heads to be higher than their stomachs to help with reflux and gas. You may also utilize a twin nursing pillow which would allow your babies to be close to you while you feed them or strap them into their car seats while they eat.

It's important to note that a baby should never be left sleeping or unattended in their car seat while it is not safely locked in the car. The way car seats rest on the floor vs the car seat dock leaves your baby at an unsafe angle that does not promote proper breathing. Also, propped feeding (where you prop a bottle up under your child) is heavily discouraged due to risk of suffocation. All babies should be closely supervised while eating.

If breastfeeding is the choice you make for yourself and your babies, then the best way to see success is to enlist support, especially if your twins are your first children. Breastfeeding is convenient and less expensive than formula and has numerous benefits for both you and your babies. Your milk has antibodies that are specifically tailored to your babies and is full of nutrients that boost brain development and their immune systems. While breastfeeding is natural and instinctive, it can take a little bit of time and effort to get it down right. I feel like this doubly true with twins. A lactation specialist can walk you through any questions or concerns you have and will watch you and your babies to ensure you are both going at it correctly.

My midwife knew that I desired to breastfeed, so before we were released to go home, she made sure both babies were latching well. Even though I had breastfed my first child, it was nice to ensure that things would continue smoothly with my twins, as every baby is different. Sometimes a lip or tongue tie can keep a baby from latching correctly, which can lead to pain for the mother or lack of milk transfer. These are issues that need to be addressed fairly quickly, both for you and your baby's sake, so if your doctor or midwife is offering this support shortly after birth, it will help with your ultimate goal of breastfeeding. Bear in mind that you do not start producing milk until two to three days after birth. What your body is producing in the meantime is colostrum, which is highly nutritious and full of needed antibodies for your babies. Your babies will not starve before your milk comes in, as their stomachs are about the size of a marble in the first few days, and colostrum is more than enough to satisfy them.

When it comes to latching, your baby's mouth will open wide to receive the nipple and surrounding areola. Milk is dispersed not solely through the nipple, but through little holes all throughout your areola nearest the nipple. Your baby's mouth should encompass most of this area, and not just the nipple itself. A correct latch should leave your baby with their lips pursed out. Babies are incredibly instinctive when it comes to eating, and most need little encouragement to latch onto the breast, but they may need a little help to get a good latch. A good latch, in my opinion, is one in which baby is comfortable, mom is comfortable, and milk is being transferred. Some will tell you there is a right or wrong way to breastfeed, but I feel like as long as these three needs are being met, you're on the right track.

Breastfeeding, while at first can be slightly uncomfortable, should not be overly painful. Sometimes pain in breastfeeding is caused by a bad latch, or baby's position. It may be necessary at times to gently break your baby's latch and try to get them repositioned. Their bodies should be facing yours, with their mouth level with your nipple. If your baby is turned out too much and having to turn their head to receive your breast, it can affect their latch.

Aside from the basics of latching, there are a few tricks and tips that help with nursing two babies at once. If this is your first-time breastfeeding, it might be helpful to start out breastfeeding one baby at a time instead of diving straight into tandem feedings. This makes the time you spend nursing a little longer but will help you get a solid grip on the basics without the frustration of juggling two hungry babies at once. Plus, it lets you see if either baby has any issues with latch.

Once you have successfully figured out how to breastfeed them individually, and you want to try feeding them together, I suggest you invest in a breastfeeding pillow specifically designed for twins. These are fairly easy to find online and can even be purchased used through your local moms of multiples group. My twin breastfeeding pillow helped me get my babies settled in comfortably so I could have my hands free to eat, drink, or help adjust their latch as needed.

My method was to get comfortable on the couch, bed, or floor, then bring each baby up onto the pillow, with their legs toward my back and their heads together at my breasts. Once they were settled, I released the boobs and then gently guided each baby to my nipples and made sure they were latched well. It may help to have your partner on hand the first few feedings as you try to navigate through this. They can hand you a baby as you get started or remove a baby that is done feeding. An extra set of hands is always helpful, though you will be amazed at how quickly you get used to doing this on your own. There are many different positions for nursing twins, and you may have to try a few before finding one that works for you.

While it is a bit trickier to breastfeed both babies at once, it does save a bit of time as well as help keep both babies on the same schedule. It's important that you make sure to alternate sides every feeding so that each baby can nurse from each breast. This helps with their eye coordination and can help encourage optimal milk production.

In the beginning you will be nursing quite a bit, so be prepared to feel like it is an around-the-clock job. Some books or experts will tell you that babies will need to eat every two to three hours, but none of my children read these books and as a result wanted to be on the breast almost every hour.

If you find yourself in a similar situation, do not stress that your babies are not getting enough milk, or that you are somehow doing it "wrong" because your precious child is not following the guidelines. It has been my experience that most breastfed babies want to nurse more frequently than what "they" say. Sometimes it's for the milk, sometimes I think it's just from the comfort of being close to Mom. Either way, breastfeeding on demand (following your baby's ques and breastfeeding whenever they want versus following a strict schedule) has its benefits for you too. It helps with ensuring you have a good milk supply, as your body produces milk on a supply-and-demand basis. Since you have two babies nursing, your body will quickly adjust to the demand. This may cause you to be quite ravenous, as making milk requires a lot of calories, which is why I highly suggest you keep water and snacks at hand while your babies nurse. It is important that you continue giving your body good nutrition while you are breastfeeding.

Overall, it can be an adjustment but nursing two babies is absolutely doable. I found breastfeeding to be a beautiful part of motherhood and I cherished the bond it created. It can be a lot of work at the beginning, but once you have it down, it can be a quick and easy solution to meal times.

If you set your mind to it and utilize the resources and support available, I believe you will find breastfeeding success.

Sleep Arrangements:

When I was pregnant, for reasons still unknown to me that I blame mostly on hormones, I was insistent that we get the twin's room set up and ready to go as soon as possible. We decorated, choose colors and themes. We bought two adorable matching cribs with matching moon-covered sheets…that neither one of my twins ever slept in.

What I didn't factor in when insisting that we have the nursery set up and ready to go was that there were two babies. Nursing them to sleep in the rocking chair before laying them in their cribs was not going to work like it had with my first child. Namely because there were two of them. We couldn't all three safely and comfortably fit in the rocking chair. Nor would I be able to gently lay one down into their crib one-handed.

We had to find another solution. What worked for one child just wasn't going to work for the others, and somehow this feels like a great revelation of parenthood. When it came to getting our twins to bed at night, I found that the best solution was a two-parent approach. My husband would get the toddler to bed while I nursed the twins, then he and I would each take a baby and gently rock or sway them to sleep. Once they were asleep, we wouldn't put them in their cribs because I (the lady who insisted on having the cribs in the first place) felt that was simply too far away. Besides, they were just going to wake up in an hour or two and want more milk anyway, so might as well keep them close by and save ourselves two trips into their room. Our solution was a smaller crib right beside our bed, much like a bassinet or co-sleeper bed.

I have to admit, for me and our needs, it was a perfect solution. We tend to be more of a co-sleeping family anyway, and having the twins close to me throughout the night allowed me to get a little more rest than I feel like I would have had otherwise.

When one twin awoke, I would pull them into bed with me and I would doze a bit while twin A got their milk. When twin B would wake to nurse, I would find that twin A was usually asleep again, so I would put twin A back in the crib, get twin B and once again doze while twin B nursed. In the event that both babies woke up at the same time, I would recline back and using the help of my husband, get each baby situated in the crooks of my arms so they could nurse while I rested. After they were done nursing, I'd put each one back into the crib.

This system met our needs perfectly. I was getting a fair amount of sleep and never really felt sleep deprived, and my babies were right beside me in a secure and separate crib. Sure, I was waking up a little more often during the night than I previously had been but since I was simply leaning over and retrieving or replacing a baby before quickly falling back asleep, it wasn't as disruptive as it would have been had I been getting up and going to the nursery multiple times a night.

Co-sleeping is a wonderful thing if done correctly. Studies have shown that babies tend to sleep better and with less stress if they are close to their mother. Babies that are close at hand can easily and quickly be soothed back to sleep before truly waking up which means more sleep for everyone. It also helps establish a good milk supply if you are nursing and studies have shown that infants that sleep in close proximity to their parents have a reduced risk of SIDS. You can practice co-sleeping without bedsharing. The two at times are used interchangeably, but they are separate practices. Bedsharing is when a baby sleeps in the same bed as the parents with no separate, designated sleeping spot of their own. Bedsharing is typically not advised for babies younger than six months old, and I personally wouldn't recommend it's use for twins. There is an increased possibility of one of the babies crawling or rolling off the bed. Co-sleeping is slightly different in that your babies are separate from your bed, in my case they had their crib right beside me, and they were only pulled into our bed when they needed to nurse.

There are some safety guidelines that you must put into place if co-sleeping or bedsharing is something you choose to do. If you take any kind of drugs or alcohol before bed, your child should never be in bed with you. Nor should you practice bedsharing if you are a particularly heavy sleeper or are prone to sleep-walking. Pillows, heavy blankets and soft-topped mattresses are not safe for babies to sleep on as they pose suffocation hazards. A firm mattress is the safest choice, so if you anticipate bringing your twins into your bed to nurse it's important to remove anything that may pose a hazard. Also, your baby should never be placed on the outside of the bed where they could crawl or roll off, nor should there be any gaps between the mattress and frame or the mattress and headboard.

I can't speak for sleep-training twins, or really any other methods of sleeping arrangements since we found what worked for us early on. However, as a parent, you know what your instincts and comfort levels are. It may take a bit of time to figure out the best arrangement for your family, but I think it's important to use common sense and do what feels right for you.

Venturing out with your hands full:

In the weeks following birth, your physical recuperation and emotional adjustment to life is of the utmost importance. However, cabin fever is a real thing and you may find yourself longing to leave the comfort of home sooner rather than later, if only to get some fresh air.

When it comes to venturing out of the house for the first time, I recommend that you start small. Perhaps a walk around the block or through your neighborhood if you feel up to it. Starting small and close to home can help give you a bit of confidence before jumping straight out into the general public.

I always recommend that you keep a fully stocked diaper bag by the door. This makes leaving for an outing so much less stressful and cuts down on the likelihood of forgetting something important. Babies love an opportunity to catch you off guard and tend to blow out their diapers the minute you get outside a five-mile radius from home. I kept my bag loaded with diapers, wipes, hand sanitizer, extra onesies, pacifiers, snacks, water, blankets, burp rags, and a plastic bag for any dirty clothes. If you are bottle feeding, it might be wise to have extra bottles and formula in your bag as well. Having our diaper bag ready at all times made me feel a little extra put together in the early days, when I mostly didn't feel put together at all.

On your first outing, it might help if you have a close friend or partner with you. They can be an extra hand if one or both babies get fussy or hungry. The stimulation of being outside or in a new place can be taxing on them, and it's important to keep in mind while your babies are small that outings should be kept relatively short. It helps if you can schedule outings around feedings or naptimes. This will help ensure that they are in better moods while you browse the grocery store. As your twins get older, they will get better at handling longer and longer forays out of the house.

Another trick to leaving the house with twin newborns that I cannot recommend enough is babywearing. I love wearing my babies. The proximity to mom seems to keep them calm while faced with new sights, smells, and sounds, plus it leaves your hands free. There are so many options for tandem babywearing, and many tutorials across the internet that can help you decide what might be best for you. You may need to practice a few different ones before you find one that works for your needs and desires. Some baby wearing groups on Facebook have local meet-ups that allow moms to try on different wearers and carriers, so that might be worth looking into before making an investment. Also, know that what works in the beginning may not work long term as your twins get bigger.

When my twins were newborns, I wrapped them in a soft stretchy wrap like a Moby or Boba. It kept them tucked close to me, and each other, and more often than not they snoozed through most early outings. The stretchy wraps are very easy to use once you get the hang of it. Once they began getting too big for the Boba, I switched to a woven wrap. Woven wraps are a bit more complex and takes a little more patience and practice to master, but they are sturdier and better equipped at handling the weight of two babies. Learning to wrap two babies to my chest with a woven wrap was definitely a skill that was extremely beneficial to have. After they outgrew the woven wrap, I used the TwinGo soft structured baby carrier. It has a bit of a price tag, but I used the carrier both at home and in public, and I daresay we got our money's worth fifteen times over. This carrier was my go-to when I needed to cook or clean, and one (or both) of my babies wanted to be held close to me, and the fact that it could be used with one or both babies was a huge perk. It also came in handy when we were trying to get one (or both) twins to sleep. Dim lights, soft noises, and a bit of swaying would usually do the trick.

Wearing my babies brought me so much confidence when I needed to leave the house with all three children by myself. It made park dates, grocery stores, and errand running so much simpler. Another perk of wearing my babies was that very few people tried to invade our personal space. I wasn't terribly concerned about germs or strangers trying to touch our babies' hands or faces, mainly because they were tucked so close to my chest.

When it comes to baby wearing, it is very important that you follow all weight recommendations and instructions for your chosen carrier/wearer. You want to make sure that your babies heads and necks are always supported, and their face is turned outward enough that they can breathe easily. Baby wearing is a safe and practical option that can make your life a little bit easier as you brave the world beyond your home.

Finding your stride:

As you settle into a routine, you gain traction into a rhythm of what does and does not work for you. Schedules get made, one day at a time, and as the days go by you start to feel less overwhelmed and a little more confident. You realize, day by day, that you are somehow making it through and slowly, you adjust to your new normal.

For every moment of rest I took during my twin pregnancy, I made up for it exponentially once my babies were born. I feel like I hit the ground running and haven't slowed down yet. There is no doubt that twins require so much work and some days it will seem endless, especially if your twins are not your first children. However, this is the life of a mother. You give everything you can to your children. When you think you can't give anymore or make it one more day, well, those are the days that you will have to dig deep into who you are to find that strength. Because let's face it, if you've made it this far, you are without a doubt an incredibly strong woman.

For now, focus on today. Just get through today and know that tomorrow will be better. You will find your stride; that sweet spot of a rhythm that makes you feel a little bit like Superwoman. It took me about two months, a ton of tears and a lot of help from my husband, friends and family, but we finally made it to a place where I felt like I could breathe.

Speaking of help, if you have it through friends, family or a hired nanny, that is amazing, and you should take advantage of every single bit of it. If friends offer to bring you cooked food or run by the grocery store for anything you need, please take them up on it. They would not offer if they did not truly care to help in some way.

Asking, or accepting help, may not be something that comes naturally to you, but I have learned that when it is offered the best thing you can do is graciously say yes, please, and thank you. I had no family nearby, no money to afford a nanny, and my husband went back to work when my twins were two weeks old. Needless to say, the first few weeks of trying to take care of my newborn twins and almost two-year-old toddler all by myself were so rough. I truly needed all the help I could get.

I feel like it was in these times of vulnerability that I truly saw the best in people. Sure, there were a lot of comments and questions from people I didn't know, but there was also so much kindness and compassion. Those early days were filled with uplifting words and well wishes, and I am still amazed at the amount of help I was constantly being offered.

One day I was leaving Costco with a cart loaded high with groceries. My twins were strapped to my chest, and I was pushing the cart with one hand while holding onto my oldest son with my other. Two men were walking toward me into the store, and upon seeing me, they immediately said "We'll load your groceries for you." And they followed me to my truck and loaded everything up.

I am so humbled and grateful to say that this wasn't a one-off case. I've completely lost track of the number of times a helping hand was lent to me, but I can honestly say that I was filled with gratitude each time. Whether it was a sympathetic smile, or an offer to return my shopping cart, or someone reaching for the item on the top shelf that I couldn't quite grasp. There was kindness and love all around me, and I was honored to see such a wonderful side of humanity. I can't help but think that I might have missed it all had it not been for the little bit of magic that twins can bring to your life.

Most of all in these coming months, go easy on yourself. Just as you allowed yourself to feel your emotions while pregnant, allow yourself to feel all your emotions while surviving this new season of life. Feel guilty if you need to when you can't soothe your babies fast enough and their cries escalate to something near inhuman. Feel exhausted and stretched thin when you're up all night trying to diaper, feed, and rock them to sleep in a never-ending cycle because *twins*. Learn to go with the flow and cut yourself some slack for the ways in which you don't feel enough. Allow yourself many moments of grace as you learn to juggle your new reality, and know that whatever you are feeling, there are moms out there who have felt it all too. Take time for yourself as you need to and try not to feel guilty at the need for a break. It takes a village and it takes a tribe, and I sincerely hope you find both. Just know that the days when it feels too hard to even keep going will one day be nothing more than a blip on the radar. These newborn days will pass quickly, and then they will be off running, and, in true twin fashion, it will likely be in opposite directions.

The most common phrase I received after I had my twins (and honestly still receive to this day) is the rhetorical (I think?) question of "how do you do it?" My standard response is a quip about pure love and caffeine. It isn't too far from the truth. Your love for your babies will supersede your anxiety. It will be greater than the fear that you can't do it, or that you aren't doing it right. It will outshine the stress and make mere shadows of your exhaustion. It will humble your pride, check your ego, and allow you to graciously say yes, please and thank you. Your love for these little souls will be your guiding light both now and in the years to come.

My advice to any new mother, especially a new mother to twins, is to listen to your instincts. There are so many books and experts telling you what to do, when to do it, how to do it, and why you should do it. However,

I have found that my heart knows what to do. It knows my babies better than anyone in the world. Your heart will guide you on this twisting, beautiful, exhausting path that is motherhood. Your instincts will know what the right choices are for you and your babies, and if you listen to your heart, you can't go wrong. Mother's intuition is a powerful thing. You were given the gift of twins. They were made from you, for you. Never doubt, for even one moment, that you are the perfect woman for this job.

I wish you all the best on this wonderful new journey. It only gets better from here.

BreAnn Blehm

Acknowledgments:

First, I have to thank my husband for not only believing in me and encouraging me through every chapter of this book, but for happily entertaining our children so I could get a moment's peace. William - you are an amazing father and partner and I could not do this life without you. Thank you for your support and thank you for manifesting this beautiful family of ours. I treasure you more than you will ever know.

To Ollie - you are my beautiful, smart, vibrant little boy. I could not be more proud of you for being you. You've had a tough gig being the big brother to twin siblings, but you handle this load so well. You are loving, kind and I am in awe of you. You made me a mother and I will forever be better for it.

To Henry & Thea - you two made our little family complete with your laughter, love, intelligence, and fiery personalities. You bring light and joy to this world and it is better because of you. You two made me a twin mother and showed me just how strong I really was, and I will forever be grateful for that gift.

To Mom and Dad - you have believed in me since I was a kid. Neither of you have ever doubted my passion or talent, and I am so grateful that you have always shown so much support for my writing. You have been an endless source of love, support, and encouragement no matter what I've tackled in this life, and I am the woman I am now because of you. I can never thank you enough for all that you do for me and my family. Thank you for believing in me. Thank you for reading my book, embracing my vision, and being there every step of the way.

To my Mama Tribe - it takes a village to raise a child, but it takes a tribe to raise a mother. You ladies are truly a gift to my life, and I am eternally grateful for the love, support, and commiseration I find in our circle. I am honored to be raising my children alongside women who are compassionate, strong, and empowering. I truly could not survive the playground, splash pad, zoo, or jump park without your willingness to be my village. Thanks for having my back.

To Kim Daly - I will be forever grateful that I found you in 2014. Throughout my pregnancies, you were an amazing source of encouragement and support, and I am so honored to have brought all my children into this world with you by my side. You are so much more than a midwife to me. You are a strong and empowered woman who has such an amazing vision for empowering other women, and my transition to motherhood and life as a mother would not be the same if not for you and the incredible community of mothers that you have created. Thank you.

Special Acknowledgements:

Front Cover Photo by Aly Renee Birth Photography

Author Photo by Kirstie Perez Photography (KPP)

Sources:

1. <u>A genome wide linkage scan for dizygotic twinning in 525 families of mothers of dizygotic twins.</u> Painter JN, Willemsen G, Nyholt D, Hoekstra C, Duffy DL, Henders AK, Wallace L, Healey S, Cannon-Albright LA, Skolnick M, Martin NG, Boomsma DI, Montgomery GW. Hum Reprod. 2010 Jun;25(6):1569-80. doi: 10.1093/humrep/deq084. Epub 2010 Apr 8.
2. American College of Obstetricians and Gynecologists. Mulitples: When It's Twins, Triplets, or More. <u>https://www.acog.org/-/media/Womens-Health/Multiples-When-Its-Twins-Triplets-or-More.pdf?dmc=1&ts=20180602T1839361322</u>
3. <u>Dietary Reference Intakes: The Essential Guide to Nutrient Requirements</u>. 2006. Institute of Medicine; Otten, Jennifer J. Hellwig, Jennifer Pitzi. Meyers, Linda D.
4. <u>Optimal Nutrition for Improved Twin Pregnancy Outcomes</u>. Goodnight, William M.D. Newman, Roger M.D. Department of Obstetrics and Gynecology, University of North Carolina, Chapel Hill, NC, USA.
5. <u>Nutrition and Multiple Gestation</u>. Luke, Barbara
6. <u>Assessing a Tool for Self-Monitoring Hydration Using Urine Color in Pregnant and Breastfeeding Women: A Cross-Sectional, Online Survey.</u> 2017. Riguad, M. Sevalho Corcao, C. Perrier, ET. Boesen-Mariani, S.

7. What are proteins and what do they do? Genetics Home Reference. NIH US National Library of Medicine. May 2018.

8. The Brewer Medical Diet for Normal and High-Risk Pregnancy. 1983. Brewer, Dr. Thomas H. Brewer, Gail Sforza. http://drbrewerpregnancydiet.com/id32.html

9. What to Expect When You're Expecting. 1984. Murkoff, Heidi. Mazel, Sharon.

10. What are Proteins? https://ghr.nlm.nih.gov/primer/howgeneswork/protein

11. Study of urine color as means of diagnosing hydration level: https://www.ncbi.nlm.nih.gov/pubmed/28614810

12. Pregnancy Nutrition: http://americanpregnancy.org/pregnancy-health/pregnancy-nutrition/

13. United States Department of Agriculture DRI Nutrient Reports: https://www.nal.usda.gov/fnic/dri-nutrient-reports

14. Prediction of Safe and Successful Vaginal Twin Birth. 2011. Breathnach FM. McAuliffe FM. Geary M, Daly S, Higgins JR, Dornan J, Morrison JJ, Burke G, Higgins S, Dicker P, Manning F, Carroll S, Malone FD; Perinatal Ireland Research Consortium. Royal College of Surgeons in Ireland, Dublin, Ireland.

15. Planned Caesarean section for Women with a Twin Pregnancy. 2015. Hofmeyr, GJ. Barrett, JF. Crowther, CA. Walter Sisulu University, University of the Witwatersrand, Eastern Cape Department of Health, East London, South Africa.

16. Neonatal Outcomes of Twin Pregnancy According to the Planned Mode of Delivery. 2008. Schmitz, T. Carnavalet, CC. Azria, E. Cabrol,

D. Goffinet, F. Maternité Port-Royal, Hôpital Cochin, AP-HP, Paris, France.

17. Management of Twins: Vaginal or Cesarean Delivery? 2015. Bibbo, C. Robinson, JN. Brigham and Women's Hospital, Boston, Massachusetts.

18. The Webster Technique: A chiropractic technique with obstetric implications. Pistolese, Richard. 2002. Journal of Manipulation and Physiological Therapeutics.

19. Tully, Gail. Spinning Babies. https://spinningbabies.com/learn-more/baby-positions/twins/

20. Pregnancy and labor massage. 2010. Field, Tiffany Ph.D. NCBI.nlm.nih.gov/pmc/articles/PMC2870995. Touch Research Institute, University of Miami School of Medicine, Florida, USA.

21. Prenatal Massage http://americanpregnancy.org/pregnancy-health/prenatal-massage/

22. New Zealand Study of Acupuncture: https://www.ncbi.nlm.nih.gov/pubmed/29482798

23. Zehra, Nihal Dolgun. Cihan, Inan. Ahmet, Salih Altintas. Preterm Labor in Twin Birth. https://www.ncbi.nlm.nih.gov/pmc/articles/PMC5017103/

24. Twin-to-Twin Transfusion Syndrome Foundation. Dr. Julian De Lia. https://www.tttsfoundation.org/.

25. Chiossi, G. Quigley, MR. Esaka, EJ. Novic, K. Celebrezze, JU. Golde, SH. Thomas, RL. Nutritional Supplementation in Monochorionic Diamniotic Twin Pregnancies; Impact on Twin-to-Twin-Transfusion

Syndrome. American Journal of Perinatology. Thieme Medical Publishers. 2008. https://www.ncbi.nlm.nih.gov/pubmed/18942043.

26. Ananth, Cande V. Smulian, John C. Demissie, Kitaw. Vintzileos, Anthony M. Knuppel, Robert A. Placental Abruption among Singleton and Twins birth in the US. American Journal of Epidemiology. V153, Issue 8, 2001.

27. Midwifery Today. Power of the Placenta. https://midwiferytoday.com/mt-articles/the-power-of-placenta/

28. Enning, Cornelia. Placenta: The Gift of Life. The Role of the Placenta in Different Cultures and How to Prepare and Use It As Medicine. 2011.

29. Complication of Multiple Pregnancy. https://www.urmc.rochester.edu/encyclopedia/content.aspx?ContentTypeID=85&ContentID=P08021

30. Frass, Kaima A. Alexandria Journal of Medicine. Vol 51, Issue 4. December 2015. Observational Study: Postpartum hemorrhage is related to hemoglobin levels in labor.

Made in the USA
Las Vegas, NV
05 February 2023

66947008R00090